TAO
AND
T'AI CHI
KUNG

TAO
AND
T'AI CHI
KUNG

ROBERT C. SOHN

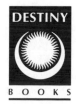

DESTINY BOOKS
ROCHESTER, VERMONT

Destiny Books
One Park Street
Rochester, Vermont 05767
www.gotoit.com

Library of Congress Cataloging-in-Publication Data
Sohn, Robert C.
    Tao and T'ai Chi Kung / by Robert C. Sohn.
      p.   cm.
    Bibliography: p.
    Includes index.
    ISBN 0-89281-217-6 (pbk.)
    1. T'ai chi ch'üan. 2. Taoism I. Title
GV504.S64 1989
613.7'1 – dc19   88-30007
                                                           CIP

Printed and bound in the United States

10 9 8 7 6 5 4

Text design by Sushila Blackman

Destiny Books is a division of Inner Traditions International

Distributed to the book trade in Canada by Publishers Group West (PGW), Toronto
Distributed to the book trade in the United Kingdom by Deep Books, London
Distributed to the book trade in Australia by Gemcraft Books, Burwood
Distributed to the book trade in New Zealand by Tandem Press, Auckland
Distributed to the book trade in South Africa by Alternative Books, Ferndale

Contents

NOTE ON CHINESE TERMS

Various English transliterations of Chinese words will often be found to represent different and important ideas. A case in point is the Chinese transliteration for the English words *energy, limit,* and *will.* The sound of all three words in Chinese is *chee.* The word for energy is often transliterated *chi* in books on T'ai Chi Chuan, however, the *chi* in T'ai Chi Chuan means limit. This kind of problem arises from the fact that as many as 400 different Chinese ideograms are pronounced with the same sound. One need only look in an English-Chinese dictionary to discover this simple fact. Some definitions in this book may conflict with the readers notion of what the word means. Please remember the 400-to-one ratio of ideas to sound and the problem will melt away. When the same sound expresses more than one idea in this book, different spellings are used; the term is defined on first usage. Specifically, *chi* means limit, *ch'i* means will, and *Qi,* after the common practice in books on Acupuncture, means "energy." (See the Appendix for a more detailed discussion of the challenges presented by translating Chinese texts.)

PREFACE

*T'*AI CHI KUNG SYMBOLIZES the ideal transformation of body and spirit into a potent, unified existence. The first step toward T'ai Chi Kung is T'ai Chi Chuan, a discipline of body expressed through form. But even this first step has its own first step: the mind must grasp the eternal principles at the root of correct movement, the stillnesses that manifest in motion. This is the Tao. By uniting these principles with disciplined movement, *Tao and T'ai Chi Kung* teaches a path for the student to follow toward enlightenment.

I am not sure when I was first introduced to the term T'ai Chi Kung, but I have used it over many years now to express the idea of the practice of spiritual enlightenment, or the perfection of the manifest reality in its individual expressions. Had any of my Chinese friends in the martial arts, most of whom are also involved in spiritual practices, questioned my use of the term, I would have probably told them I made it up. They, however, seemed immediately clear about my meaning. It's interesting that the term is conspicuously absent from the vocabulary of all my Occidental friends in the martial arts.

The use of the term Kung Fu to mean "Chinese martial arts" is one of the great errors of modern American usage in this field. In fact, Chinese martial arts are properly called "Wu Shu" and are divided into "inner power" and "outer power" schools, call Nei Chia and Wu Chia, respectively. Mastery in one of these schools is either Kung Fu Nei Chia, or Kung Fu Wu Chia.

Kung means mastery or perfection. Since the T'ai Chi is the balance of Yin and Yang, then T'ai Chi Kung can mean "the perfection of balance" or "attunement with the Tao," the way that the universe is supposed to unfold. Since T'ai Chi is literally translated "Great Limit," in contrast to Wu Chi or the "Empty Limit," it refers to the Manifest Reality. It can also be translated as the "perfection of the Manifest Reality." These are different ways of expressing the idea of spiritual enlightenment.

This book is an attempt to reawaken the knowledge that T'ai Chi Chuan and T'ai Chi Qi Kung are major techniques of Taoist Yoga with potentials that extend beyond the physical level. To a large degree, the practice of Hatha Yoga exercises has been divorced from the full practice of self-development (*sadhana*) in Indian Yoga. However, the roots, the larger spiritual framework, have not been completely forgotten. This fate of isolation from spiritual roots, however, has befallen T'ai Chi Chuan. I am not a "lover of tradition" who wishes to set the record straight. I am a teacher of esoteric philosophy, and as such, I have devoted a long time to teaching the practical application of the principles of spiritual development. This has been with the end purpose of producing recognizable transformation in my pupils, to see them evolve on the path toward spiritual Self-realization. T'ai Chi Chuan, in the proper context, is a firm and powerful foundation for this spiritual development. I hope this book will open the door to a broader valuation and use of T'ai Chi Chuan in its spiritual context.

PREPARING
THE MIND
FOR
T'AI CHI
CHUAN

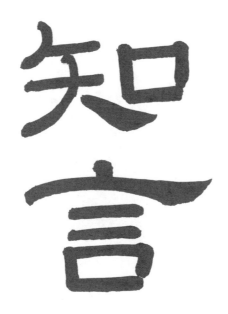

PART ONE

1

Introduction to the Fundamentals of Taoist Thought

THE FIRST RECORD OF THE tenents of Taoist philosophy is in the ostensible writings of an ancient, possibly mythical, figure called Lao Tze—an appellation meaning "the old (ancient, hoary) philosopher"—who taught the way of enlightenment twenty-five hundred years ago. He, like others who have come to teach higher ideas, had grown more and more disenchanted with the lack of results[1] despite the passage of time and the application of much effort to teach on his part. He decided to "leave the dead to bury their own dead" (Matthew 8:22) and go up into the mountains to wait in peace until time came to depart from the world. As he was leaving the city, the gatekeeper stopped him and pleaded with him to at least leave some document, some kind of information, some kind of reference to be cherished by those who sought the Way. Legend tells us that the old philosopher then composed the Book of the Universal Way and its Individual Reflection—the *Tao Teh Ching.*

An interesting anecdote from the classics illustrates the position of Taoist thought in the mainstream of Chinese culture. Kung Fu Tze was master of the expression of the normative basis of Chinese culture and, of course, all derivative "Confucian" cultures, as in Japan, Korea, Thailand, et al. Kung Fu Tze went to visit Lao Tze[2] and discoursed with him on philosophy. When he returned to his school, his students anxiously pressed him for a discussion of the experience. Finally the master spoke. All he would say is, "I have visited the dragon, and he ascended into the heavens where

I could not even think to follow." He would say no more. This points to the fact that, in general, Taoist thought is "transcendental" philosophy and not simple easily-grasped rules of behavior. Grasping the Taoist point of view requires the ability to evaluate conceptually and manipulate a multitude of variables leading to the unification of all ideas in the universal Tao. This is the basis of the profound thinking of the great master of strategy, Sun Tze, and also of the clearly mythical Yellow Emperor of Acupuncture fame, as well as that expressed in much of the intellectual literature that has been taken as Chinese thought. But these great works of philosophy are no more the ideas of common man in China than are the writings of Walt Whitman typical of the thought and feelings of everyday citizens of the United States. The esoteric philosophy of any nation is *not* in any way typical of national thought, and the esoteric philosophies of *all* nations are essentially the same. Taoist thought, not reduced to magic as in the common view, is an esoteric philosophy and its arts—T'ai Chi Chuan, Pau Kua Chung, and Hsing I Chuan—have both exoteric and esoteric[3] values.

The concept of Tao is the cornerstone of Taoist philosophy. The basic meaning of the Tao pictogram is a path or road. As an ideogram it further implies a path toward a goal, a method of gaining an end or a type of art. In the generally accepted view of the modern scholar, it implies the Way of the universe, the proper unfolding of what is and what is to be. "All that exists between heaven and earth is law and energy." The Tao is the unfolding universe, the interaction of energy according to law, or as it is described poetically in one of the major philosophies of India: The Absolute has an eternal aspect called *lila,* divine play, which is manifest as the interplay of the positive and negative aspects of the world—Shiva and Shakti, the eternal divine lovers. "She became a ewe, and he became a ram and coupled with her; she became a cow and he became a bull . . . thus was all created."[4]

The *Teh,* as in Tao Teh Ching, means Virtue in the ancient Greek sense of "perfection." So it is taught that when a man strives to be in accord with the Tao, his efforts will cause being transformation and he will eventually attain the state of human perfection or Teh. For the Teh of a man is the individual reflection of the Tao of the Universe. When a man has Teh, he is in tune with the Universal Tao. When he dies, he unites with the Universe. As long as he is alive the Tao reflects in him as Teh.

The ideogrammatic quality of the Chinese written language is clearly demonstrated in the symbol for Teh, Virtue 德 . As we dissect and analyze the Chinese character, the depth of its meaning should become clear. This element (彳) is the abbreviated form of the verb "to act" or "to go," implying that the character is a verb or the name of a process. This element (✛) is the symbol for the number ten, and is also, by convention, used as a sign for "strong" or "extreme." When combined with the symbol for action, it implies a "strong action," or perhaps "much effort." This symbol (▨) is a fishnet, further implying that this strong action or great effort will involve some kind of catching or enclosing. The single horizontal line in a Chinese character (━) is a convention meaning "plentifulness." This character (心) is "the heart." Thus we have a strong action (彳) of netting (limiting, controlling) the plentifulness of the heart (罒心).

What is it to limit the plentifulness of the heart? Based on Lao Tze's comment that "Ever desiring, one can see the manifestations," and on the Chinese medical principle that the "Heart harbors the human soul," it is reasonable to assume that the plentifulness of the heart is "desire," and therefore we are being told to control desire. The control of desire, which is essentially the control of the personal self, or false self (ego), is the state of Virtue or perfection. Self-control leads to the Tao.

Taoism, like all profound philosophical systems, is based on the assumption that the underlying state of reality is nothing—no-thing. Therefore, the first symbol of the Taoist creative process is an empty circle. This

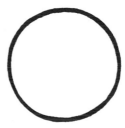

Fig. 1. The empty circle represents Wu Chi

empty circle represents Wu Chi. *Wu* means "empty" or "void"; *Chi* means "limit." Thus we have the empty limit, the final no-thing; the ultimate emptiness.

The Buddhists call the state of ultimate attainment Sunyata, the Void. In the Vedantic philosophy of India, the highest state is called Nirguna Brahman. Wu Chi and Nirguna Brahman are references to the same reality and are in fact virtually identical in translation. *Brahman* literally means "the Immense," that which is greater than the sum of all there is; it is usually translated as the Absolute. *Chi* means "the Limit," the extreme conditions of being. *Nir* means "devoid" or "empty," and *guna* means "quality." *Nirguna Brahman* means the qualityless Absolute, totally empty while yet encompassing all, devoid of any qualities. Wu Chi means the qualityless Absolute, the state in which everything is swallowed up and is nothing.

The Universe Is Manifest Through Motion

All teachings, whether scientific or philosophical, begin with the idea of an unspecified event which must have occurred so that the process of the Universe could begin. The simplest expression of this—without scientific hypotheses about energy explosions or mystical symbolism designed to evoke a sense of higher knowledge—is to say, "In the beginning, there is movement." As It is always in Its unmanifest state, It is ultimately quiescent; It is not moving, It is not active. The Gyana yogis[5] analyze the nature of the Absolute by a series of questions such as, "Is the Absolute the God Shiva?" "Neti, Neti," they answer; "It is not limited to that." When you have totally negated everything, you are left with the Void, Wu Chi. That is the Absolute. Somehow there is motion in the non-motion. The motion is the first manifestation. It is called Yang. As the motion evolves to the next limit, to the point where there is no other possibility of moving, it reverses its nature and becomes non-motion or quiescence. The quiescence, which is the limit of action, is called Yin. The movement, which is the limit of quiescence, is called Yang. These two are the same, for they are extremes of what is. The Motion and Quiescence constantly interact. There is Motion in Quiescence and Quiescence in Motion. They are interdependent ideas, as an old song said in a different age about love and marriage, "You can't have one without the other." This will *always* be true, however, of motion and quiescence (or rest). We can look briefly at the classic illustration of relativity in physics,[6] remembering to imagine as all scientists must do when they experiment, that we are not part of the Universe that we are studying. This is to remove whatever influence we may have on the studied system. Imagine one body (planet) in empty space. If we try to discover the presence or absence of motion of the planet, we discover that the question of motion is really devoid of meaning in this artificial world consisting of only one object. All our experiences of movement are, although not consciously considered to be such, relative to a place of rest. That's why people in a motionless vehicle may be momentarily startled upon noticing motion relative to another vehicle, and erroneously believe that their vehicle is in motion. Until some other body at rest is noted, the person has no way of telling which vehicle is really in motion. So we always tacitly ask the question, "What is the resting point that is the referent of the motion?" Therefore, it is necessary to introduce a second body into our very limited universe. Then it is possible to conceptualize that one body is in a state of rest and one is in motion—either body can be taken as "at rest." There is really no distinction between the two. Their relative motion exists interdependently; one cannot be considered in terms of motion without the other. Only the Ultimate Quiescence can be without motion. But that Wu Chi is beyond any experiential universe. Therefore the Yang and the Yin, the motion and the absence of motion, are essentially one thing, as our two bodies in the physics illustration have shown. The two arise together from the creative urge of the Absolute; they must exist interdependently or they cannot exist at all. Therefore when one ceases to be manifest, both have ceased. There is either Yin/Yang or there is nothing.

Purpose Is Inherent in the Wu Chi

Inevitably philosophers are plagued with the question, "Why does the Wu Chi manifest motion?" And this taunting question leaves us, no matter how much we may deliberate, with only two possible answers: either accident or intention underlies the motion. The possibility of accident in the Absolute denies the very idea of Consciousness. Indian philosophy expresses this idea by stating that the first manifestation of the Absolute is "Satchida-nanda," which is composed of the three words: *sat* (existence), *chit* (consciousness), and *ananda* (bliss). Chart 1 on page 6 shows the devolution of these primary experiences into what man calls existence, thought, and feeling in the gross material world. The particular manifestations of events in the material universe could be considered the result of the random interaction of the three constituents of the primary creation. However, the fact that *all* possibilities occur is attested to by modern science in the concept of waves of probability. This is also the position of esoteric philosophers as expressed by P.D. Ouspensky in the idea of the "5th dimension as the realm of all realized and unrealized possibilities."[7] Since all varieties of intelligence and consciousness are inevitable, the source must contain and be greater than the greatest of the possible manifestations of consciousness. This then brings us to the conclusion that there is fundamentally an intention, a purposefulness, in the very fact of the motion—that consciousness is inherent in the primary condition. This fundamental idea or notion of movement is called *li,* and the principle of *li* is the basic source of the formation of all that is. First there is a *li* of anything—a notion, an idea, a picture. Then there must be *ch'i* or "will to accomplish," and slowly it manifests as material

CHART 1. Descent or Limitation of Being

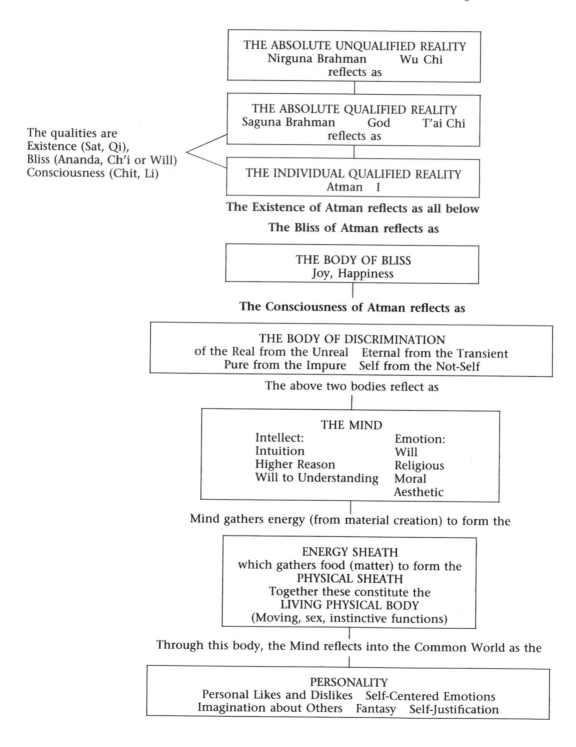

The qualities are
Existence (Sat, Qi),
Bliss (Ananda, Ch'i or Will)
Consciousness (Chit, Li)

THE ABSOLUTE UNQUALIFIED REALITY
Nirguna Brahman   Wu Chi
reflects as

THE ABSOLUTE QUALIFIED REALITY
Saguna Brahman   God   T'ai Chi
reflects as

THE INDIVIDUAL QUALIFIED REALITY
Atman   I

The Existence of Atman reflects as all below

The Bliss of Atman reflects as

THE BODY OF BLISS
Joy, Happiness

The Consciousness of Atman reflects as

THE BODY OF DISCRIMINATION
of the Real from the Unreal   Eternal from the Transient
Pure from the Impure   Self from the Not-Self

The above two bodies reflect as

THE MIND
Intellect: Emotion:
Intuition   Will
Higher Reason   Religious
Will to Understanding   Moral
                              Aesthetic

Mind gathers energy (from material creation) to form the

ENERGY SHEATH
which gathers food (matter) to form the
PHYSICAL SHEATH
Together these constitute the
LIVING PHYSICAL BODY
(Moving, sex, instinctive functions)

Through this body, the Mind reflects into the Common World as the

PERSONALITY
Personal Likes and Dislikes   Self-Centered Emotions
Imagination about Others   Fantasy   Self-Justification

occurrence in time. *Li differentiates in the "world of ideas," and this is reflected in the material universe as the constituents and the events of experiential existence.*[8]

This original great Movement and Quiescence (see Chart 2, page 11) merge into one and this One is called the T'ai Chi: the Great Limit, the Manifest Absolute, Saguna Brahman (the Absolute with qualities). These qualities are *sat-chit-ananda*—Existence, Consciousness, and Bliss.

This diagram symbolizes the concept of the T'ai Chi which is the balance between motion and motionlessness, Yin and Yang. Yang, motion, having reached its limit, is motionless, Yin. This is T'ai Chi.

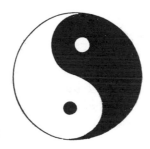

FIG. 2. Yin and Yang

T'ai Chi and Wu Chi are two extremes of the same fundamental reality. When Yang/motion and its corollary Yin/rest totally cease to be manifest, the T'ai Chi dissolves into Wu Chi. When the Yang/motion manifests, the Wu Chi appears as T'ai Chi. They are limits—one is the extreme of the other. From the Void, from the Absolute nothing, from the absence of all, there is motion. But that motion is balanced with quiescence. When quiescence reaches a limit, it becomes motion. This is an expression of an ever-existent, wave-like reality. It also expresses the Law of Three—three primary forces interacting: Yin, Yang, and the force of the Whole, the Balance, the Return. This is a creative process going from one extreme to the other, showing endless cycles of reality.

It is written that from this T'ai Chi stem the Six and from the Six appear the Five, and from the Five come the Ten Thousand Things. The Five are the five elements or Five Elemental Forces. These are not, as some modern readers often think, elements in the sense of the ninety-two elements of the Periodic Table. The five elemental forces are five types or levels of energy manifestation. The Chinese term for the energy that makes up the substance of the Universe is Qi, which should not be confused with the term *chi* (limit) and *ch'i* (will to action). These five basic forms of Qi are Fire, Earth, Metal, Water, and Wood. Metal encompasses mineral, hydrogen, and other elements. Wood encompasses plant life. Plant life is literally rooted to the earth, grows from the earth, and is constantly alive in one form or another in the earth. Wood, therefore, becomes the symbol of life. The Fire element encompasses heat, light, the digestive process, anger, and so on. Water encompasses all liquid forms, as well as yielding to force. And the Earth is the center, the balancer of all the other forces, the sustainer of life. For example, the spleen and stomach, which are concerned with the basic life-sustaining function of digestion and assimilation in the body, are considered Earth in Chinese medicine. Thus, all that there is in the universe can be categorized into five elemental energy manifestations, by taking the qualities of the object considered and recognizing that qualitative relationship to the Five Principles. The Six cannot be so easily categorized in the material world for they refer to more subtle levels of universal energies. They categorize the qualities of Yin and Yang as great Yin, balanced Yin, diminishing Yin, great Yang, bright Yang and diminished Yang. Since all the Qi of the channels is one or another of these qualities, this is important in Chinese medical diagnosis, but has little other practical value. The Ten Thousand Things is a reference to the material world.

First Chapter of the Tao Teh Ching

Now we will look at the *Tao Teh Ching,* the Book of the Way and the Virtue, as translated by Gia-fu Feng. The first chapter begins:

> *The Tao that can be told is not the eternal Tao.*
> *The name that can be named is not the eternal name.*
> *The nameless is the beginning of Heaven and Earth.*
> *The named is the mother of the Ten Thousand Things.*
> *Ever desireless, one can see the mystery.*
> *Ever desiring, one can see the manifestations.*
> *These two spring from the same source but differ in name;*
> *this appears as darkness.*
> *Darkness within darkness. The gate to all mystery.*

This explains succinctly all of Taoist philosophy: the creation process, the final result of that process and the kind of work that must be done to accomplish the purpose of existence, which is to re-experience the pre-creation state.

CHART 2. Devolution from the Wu Chi

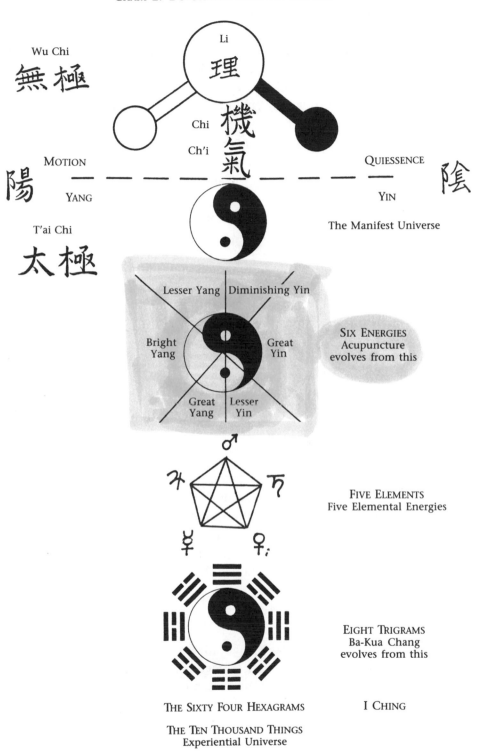

Wu Chi
無極

Li
理

Chi
Ch'i

機氣

MOTION
陽
YANG

QUIESSENCE
陰
YIN

The Manifest Universe

T'ai Chi
太極

Lesser Yang | Diminishing Yin

Bright
Yang

Great
Yin

Great
Yang

Lesser
Yin

SIX ENERGIES
Acupuncture
evolves from this

FIVE ELEMENTS
Five Elemental Energies

EIGHT TRIGRAMS
Ba-Kua Chang
evolves from this

THE SIXTY FOUR HEXAGRAMS   I CHING

THE TEN THOUSAND THINGS
Experiential Universe

The Tao that can be told is not the eternal Tao.

All of our communication relates to the "T'ai Chi" and its manifestations. There is nothing that can be said of the Void. That is the ultimate Tao, the ultimate Reality, the ultimate Way. The Tao that can be told is not the eternal Tao. What can we say about the Void? Nothing.

The name that can be named is not the eternal name.

Whatever we name about the Ten Thousand Things, the Five Elements, the T'ai Chi, Yin and Yang, is not eternal. They are ephemeral; they pass in and out of existence, endlessly. All that is eternal cannot be named: emptiness, Wu, nothing.

The nameless is the beginning of Heaven and Earth.

The nameless is what we call the Empty Limit—Wu Chi. That appellation could be seen as a name, but it is like naming a thing, "thing." It is, rather than a name, a method of pointing toward an idea. This is the beginning of Heaven and Earth, Yang and Yin. The primary manifestations of Yang and Yin are Heaven and Earth. When the Sunyata or the Void moves, there is activity—Yang or Heaven; the initial creative process from the first reality down through the various levels of manifestation. Finally, at the end is Earth, the ultimate Yin.[9] So Heaven is the shining, the energetic. As it moves down it becomes less and less Yang, until it finally becomes Yin, the dark, the end, the terminus of action; the quiescence in the other extreme. The Sunyata is the quiescence that contains everything. The Earth is the quiescence which is dense and has no substance other than its own denseness. So, Heaven and Earth are Yang and Yin. The Sunyata, the Void, the Wu Chi, the nameless, is the beginning of Heaven and Earth. Heaven and Earth are T'ai Chi, the whole of reality, Yang and Yin interacting.

The named is the mother of the Ten Thousand Things.

The named is Heaven and Earth, T'ai Chi. From the interaction of Yang and the Yin, there manifests the Five Elements. Finally the manifest universe results from the interaction of the Yang and the Yin, Heaven and Earth.
Then comes the summary of the great work of Taoism.

Ever desireless, one can see the mystery.

If an aspirant of Eternal Truth has conquered his worldly nature by subduing and conquering the passion and desire of life, and has focused his being through development of body, mind, and emotions, thereby coming into the state of harmony in all his centers, he has attained the state of desirelessness. Such a being can comprehend the true reality that is obscured by the world of illusion produced by the continuation of desire.

Ever desiring, one can see the manifestations.

As long as objects draw the attention, as long as man's desire is not controlled, just so long will one see the manifest material universe as opposed to its underlying real source. This is not, as many like to think, a statement about morality and right behavior. It is about dissolution of any emotional bindings to the world of man's experience and refocusing the attention on the incorporeal world.

These two spring from the same source but differ in name.

The mystery (the T'ai Chi) and the manifestation (the Ten Thousand Things) spring from the same source, but differ in name. The source is Wu Chi, nothingness, emptiness. Ultimately, that is reality. The T'ai Chi is the balance of the whole of manifestation and is the manifest reality that we seek to experience, while the Ten Thousand Things is the fragmented, linear, time-bound manifest reality that we do experience—yet they are the same. The understanding of their sameness is a very important step toward the understanding of T'ai Chi Kung. Only the unmanifest is the real, and only the T'ai Chi is its perfect reflection. Just so, to the newly awakening mind within the level of the Ten Thousand Things, only the T'ai Chi is real, and the world of experience is its reflection. The beginning of the *Iso-Upanishad* reads "Om, that is perfect, this is perfect. This is a perfect reflection of that. Remove the perfect reflection and the underlying perfection remains."[10]

Darkness within darkness. The gate to all mystery.

The gate to all mystery is Teh. The attainment or practice of Teh seems like a meaningless and pointless activity to those who are bound by darkness and ignorance. Those who seek the Way are often seen as ignorant by worldly men. Yet it is the world of illusion that is indeed Darkness. What appears as Darkness to worldly men is in fact the Light which they cannot comprehend: "And the light shined in the darkness, but the Darkness comprehended it not."[11]

The Yin and the Yang

We have thus far explained the material manifestation: how it "moves" from ultimate nothingness, from the reality which we refer to as the Void, to the manifest universe. One manifests two, Motion and Quiescence, Yang and Yin. Yang is vibration, pulse, movement; the world is vibration, pulse, movement—varying forms of "energy," all interacting against a background of varying forms of Yin, or rest, that tempers the power of the Yang.[12] The scientific description of the world is in terms of energy changes, and what was previously called particle physics has been renamed in recent years high-energy physics. The varying changes are varying manifestations of the Yang as it is tempered by the Yin.

We must understand this as a relative concept. Compare three of the five elements: Fire, Water, Earth. Fire is clearly Yang in relation to Water and Earth. Fire is the most active, the most energetic. Earth is clearly Yin in relation to Water and Fire because it is much denser, heavier, devoid of movement. Water is Yin compared to Fire, yet Yang compared to Earth, since compared to Fire, Water is dense and devoid of movement, yet compared to Earth, Water is highly mobile. So the concepts of Yin and Yang are interdependent, relative concepts. There is no Yin without Yang; there is no Yang without Yin. You have both, otherwise you have nothing. Everything in the universe, therefore, is a manifestation of the interdependent, relative relationship between the poles of Yin and Yang. If we take a stick and designate one end of the stick complete Yang and the other end complete Yin, breaking the stick in half will leave us with two identical sticks; one end of each is complete Yang in relation to the other end of the same stick, which is complete Yin. There is no way that you can break Yin and Yang apart because the moment you do away with the Yin, you also do away with the Yang. They go together. There cannot be the one without the other. The Void, the ultimate Reality, *is,* whether it is residing in its own nature or whether it underlies the interaction of Yin and Yang.

The more Yin—the more dense, the less energetic and the more material something is; the more Yang—the lighter, the more energetic and the less dense the thing is. Thus, there is an infinite variation in the balance between Yin and Yang, there an infinite variety of manifest substances.

Everything on this Earth is interacting Yin and Yang, yet compared to anything a level above the Earth, the Earth is all Yin. The Earth is Yin; Heaven is Yang. The things of Heaven compared to each other are Yin and Yang, but compared to Earth they are all Yang.

A Discussion on the Origin of Consciousness

Let us briefly look at the materialist viewpoint, which has usually been thought to be the *scientific* idea of the evolution of consciousness. It has been held in some established Western scientific circles that consciousness is a product of unconsciousness; that a universe devoid of the qualities of thought somehow, through the aggregation of its material nature, develops the quality of thought. A universe devoid of awareness somehow, through the aggregation of material substance, develops awareness.[13]

It is very difficult to comprehend the reasoning behind such an idea. How can the higher come out of the lower? Traditional science told us that it is an accident of chemical combinations. Through experiments conducted during our required schooling, it has become well known that there is no phenomenon of spontaneous generation of life from dead matter. Yet, apparently if we allow a long, long time, then we can assume generation of life from dead matter? Even allowing the possibility of the generation of life from non-life, we are left with the question of the generation of a state of other-consciousness and self-consciousness as mental activity generated from matter. There are many in our modern world who would relegate all sentient experience, including all cognitive functions as well as mystical experiences, to the position of by-products of the activity of the physical organism. I can only suggest that such thinkers question the reason for the arising of all mental activities beyond the needs of the physical animal. Does this quality, which is claimed to not exist until it becomes manifest, have any sense or basis for arising in the context of animal existence? In fact, the spiritual and other higher mental faculties of man have become a negative force in the proper evolution of the animal species, Homo sapiens, and could not have arisen if the simplistic evolutionary viewpoint behind the rejection of primary consciousness is correct.[14] In addition, the stuff of the living body is essentially the same as the stuff of dead matter, with a strange inexplicable something which enlivens it and is beyond the measurements of Western science. Under examination, live tissue is the same (except for being alive) as dead tissue. But the "substance" of mental activity is not substance and therefore there is no substance aggregation that could generate such a phenomena.

Western science gives us a story that is not radically different from the Chinese or Hindu conception (except for the primacy of consciousness in these latter views). It is called the Big Bang theory. Once upon a time (and time is a difficult problem with ramifications beyond the scope of this text) in the "center" of the infinite universe, an infinite mass of energy was densely packed into a tiny space. For some inexplicable reason, something happened in the energy that caused it to expand infinitely into the infinite universe and, in the process of expansion, take on many different forms. These forms include living, self-generating consciousness, aware "stuff." The only difference lies in what the evolutionists find in the genes of all living things—the blueprints or modifiable plans on which each creature and general evolution is made. Taoists and all other esoteric philosophers agree as to the existence of the preexistent plan; however, it is carried back to the very Source of all that is, as expressed in the opening of the New Testament, "In the beginning was the Word, and the Word was with God . . . and without him (the Word) was not anything made." (John, 1:1-3)

Consciousness Is Intrinsic in Wu Chi

It seems clear that life—or the energetic force which is life, which is awareness, which is consciousness—must be intrinsic in the nature of reality. It must be intrinsic in the ultimate state, in the Sunyata, in the Void. There must be awareness, otherwise it cannot arise. That there would be awareness first, and nothing to be aware of, is more comprehensible than that there would be something to be aware of and nothing aware of it.

In fact, given this scheme, and given a perception of the universe as we have it now, scientifically as well as esoterically—as energy that is bound in various ways—then clearly *awareness defines the universe.* It is the way one perceives the energy that defines the universe. Without awareness, there is no universe. Try to imagine a universe without awareness. I can imagine a universe with nothing conscious *in* it, but I cannot imagine one with nothing conscious *of* it, since to imagine it requires my consciousness *of* it. But given that we are conscious of it, we define what we see, we make the universe what it is. Awareness is the foundation of the events of the material universe, according to contemporary high-energy physics. Waves of probability, not substance or events, make up what is—until some consciousness intervenes and one of the probabilities is realized. That which occurs is directly dependent on the consciousness that "invokes" the waves of probability. So we look at it this way. Again, in the beginning is Wu Chi. However, something is inherent in this Wu Chi. The Hindus describe that "something" very effectively with a story that says, "In the beginning was the Self like a person alone. And it said, 'I am afraid. But of what am I afraid? For there is no other.' Thus was other conceived."[15] This is the Vedantic poetry that attempts to give a broader emotional sense to the idea that in the beginning was the One, Brahman without attributes. Because of the intrinsic quality of awareness in this unlimited and unfragmented reality, duality must be conceived. That is, awareness seeks something else of which to be aware. This the God Shiva, *Aham,* I Am, thinking of Shakti, the Female Power, who dances and he loses himself in her, *Idam.* This is the "I" that conceives, the "Thou" of Martin Buber, the Hebrew mystic. All who see, see that in this is the T'ai Chi formed—by the Self conceptualizing other. In the Void there is conceived motion and there is motion. "God said, 'Let there be light,' and there was light" is the manner of expression of this truth in the West (Genesis 1:3).

Discussion of the Principle of Li (Notion)

The Taoists speak of the *li* of things, their reason, conception, notion. *Li* is inherent in Wu Chi. The conceptualization of the universe is primary. At first there is nothing but the idea. Then, when the idea becomes manifest as the world, the whole universe is nothing but idea and its manifestations. As the Chinese proverb says, "All that exists between Heaven and Earth is law and energy." *Li* is the idea or notion, and *ch'i* is the "will to manifestation," and resultant therefrom is Qi, or the manifest reality.

From this ultimate nothingness there is *conceived* motion and thus there is motion. The motion of Yin and Yang is perceived as six forms or qualities of Yin and Yang, and their interactions become differentiated into five fundamental material energy classifications, and from these come ten thousand different kinds of interacting things. Always, however, behind that there lies *li.* Nothing becomes manifest without first being conceived.

Plato spoke of the World of Ideas. Because there is a chair, somewhere there is a world in which there is a perfect chair, the ideal chair, the *ideal* of a chair. It is not a material chair, but rather an idea.[16] Every chair that ever exists does so only as a temporary expression of the ideal chair in Plato's World of Ideas. Every chair that ever comes into existence exists only because that concept exists. Plato explained that the quality of existence was inherent in the permanent world of ideas, and that the ideal world, being without time, is the real, while the manifest universe, being temporary, was ephemeral. The "ideal" (concept) of chair always exists. The material chair passes in and out of existence in a flash. It may be fifty years, but that is nothing in eternity. Things come and go, ideas are eternal.

Sentient beings are not quite the same. The ideal man is more real than manifest man, but on a different "plane of existence."[17] Of course, on this plane of existence, on this level of world, the only thing that has any substance is substance. But when one attunes to a different level of world, this world becomes more ephemeral, and the stuff of the other world becomes much more substantial.

Why are children born with particular physical, mental, emotional, and moral qualities? Because there is *li*. Depending on the philosophical orientation, the basic *li* will be caused by what may be called karma, causal body, time body, etc. Carl Jung called the underlying defining drives of a given human group the collective unconscious. This is the result of the history of man's forbearers expressed as a series of expectations and patterns of response in terms of observation of the world. There are notions in his belly, which includes the three lower psychic centers, or *tan tien* (see Chart 3, page 19). The *li* is printed in the genes of a child. The conceptualization of the child is carried in the genes, a set of details incomprehensibly compressed into one cell. Apparently there is energetically locked into the gene, into the cell itself, the idea of the fully developed entity. Insofar as there were not such an idea, nothing would develop.

An interesting experiment was performed by Cleve Backster, an early researcher in plant response. Backster attached an egg to a galvanometer, a device that measures small changes in electrical activity. The experiment is described in *The Secret Life of Plants:*[18]

> For nine hours Backster got an active chart recording from the egg, corresponding to the rhythm of the heartbeats of the chicken embryo, the frequency being between 160 and 170 beats per minute, appropriate to an embryo three or four days along in incubation. Only the egg was store-bought, acquired at the local delicatessen, and was unfertilized. Later, breaking the egg and dissecting it, Backster was astonished to find that it contained no

physical circulatory structure of any sort to account for the pulsation. He appeared to have tapped into some sort of force field not conventionally understood within the present body of scientific knowledge.

There was a rudimentary chicken, in a sense, an incorporeal chicken in the egg. In scientific circles, there is a growing belief that an energy body preceded the existence of the material body. Marcel Vogel, a brilliant research chemist, has worked with liquid crystals and has concluded that crystals are brought into physical existence by preforms, or ghost images, of pure energy which anticipate the solids.[19] This is similar to the concept of the energy body, which is an idea, that is, a less-material existence followed by the matter that expresses it concretely. This is closer to *li*. Of course, it is still a material thing, so that we must conceive another less material substance behind that and another one behind that; in fact, there are six levels of bodies of ever finer and less encumbered being underlying the gross material being body of mankind. This is discussed further below.

In sum, from within the Wu Chi, the ultimate Reality, there manifests *li*, ideation. From the idea, there is *ch'i*, the will to manifestation. From that will, there manifests Qi, existence, substance, matter, energy, form.

These three—*li, ch'i*, and Qi—Idea, Will and Energy/matter, correspond to the Hindu trilogy of Satchitananda—Existence, Consciousness, Bliss. Bliss and Will are the emotional nature. Consciousness is Idea, and Existence is Energy/matter.

Man as a Descent from the Absolute

The Adwaite Vedanta[20] of India is most explicit in describing the "being bodies" of man and, with some modification in terminology and emphasis, we can clearly see the process of T'ai Chi Kung.

The Absolute Reality reflects itself as three forces or powers which we have called existence, consciousness (awareness), and bliss (emotional feeling). This tripartite reality is particularized through the conceptualization of "other," and thus it is reflected as the Atman or individual Self. The Atman in its aspect as bliss reflects as the "body of bliss" which, although very pure and advanced, is but a reflection of the true Bliss. The Atman in its aspect as consciousness reflects through the body of bliss as the body of discrimination. The bodies of bliss and discrimination (as "feeling" and "thought") reflect as the mind made of the intellect and the emotions. This body (the mind), which may contain will, although capable of receiving intuitive knowledge and experiencing higher religious, moral, and aesthetic emotions, is only a reflection of the nature and abilities of higher being bodies. The mind, interacting with the world of matter, produces an energy body, which gathers to itself an aggregate of material substance in the form of food to form a gross material vehicle called a physical body. This physical body and the energy body that enlivens it is called the living physical body. This is the field of action of the work of Tai Chi Kung. The mind reflects through the physical body as the personality and the physical body become the field of action of the world. Thus the great work and the great illusion meet in the physical body.

The whole complex of being bodies from the body of bliss to the personality is a reflection of the Atman in its aspect as existence (see Chart 1, page 8).

The practice of T'ai Chi Chuan is the primary effort to draw back from the personality and become in tune with the physical and energy bodies. The practice of T'ai Chi Kung encompasses the process of pulling back again and again, until the ultimate return to the Atman and finally to the Absolute.

Each of the described being bodies has a kind of connection to the energy body according the the hermetic maxim, "As above, so below." The *tan tien,* containing the three lowest control centers of the energy body (instinctual, sexual, and motile), is the connection of the physical and energy bodies. The Heart center is the connection of the emotional aspect of the mind. The Throat center is the connection of the intellectual aspect of the mind. The Third Eye center is the connection of the body of discrimination and the Crown center is the connection of the body of bliss. Alignment of these seven centers is a constant underlying activity of T'ai Chi Kung (see Chart 3, page 21).

Practical Psychology: The Use of Li to Change Qi

The practical Chinese Taoist method of attaining enlightenment is to aid the mind to evolve deeper and more powerful *li. Li* is the underlying aspect of Qi, energy/matter. Without *li* there is no Qi. The nature of *li* defines the nature of Qi. The way the idea is, *is* the way the world is.

Qi is manifest in a multitude of forms, symbolized by concepts such as the Yin and the Yang, the Six Energies, the Five Elements, the Eight

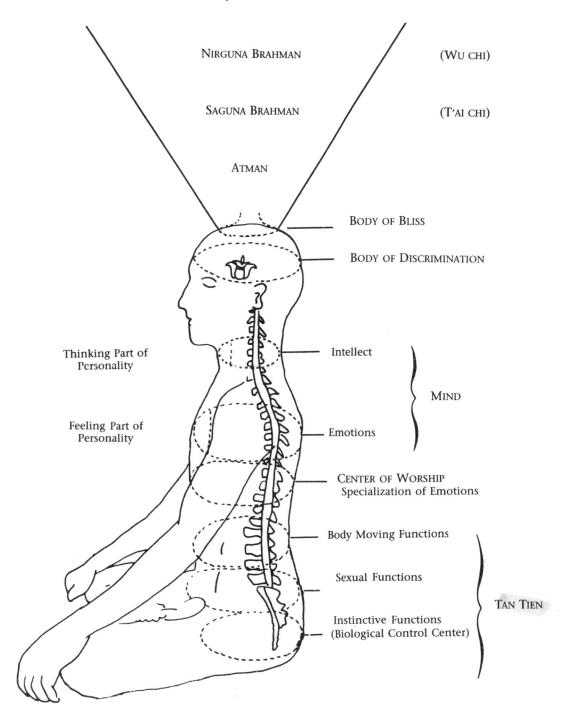

CHART 3. Psychic Centers of Man

NIRGUNA BRAHMAN   (WU CHI)

SAGUNA BRAHMAN   (T'AI CHI)

ATMAN

BODY OF BLISS

BODY OF DISCRIMINATION

Thinking Part of
Personality

Intellect

MIND

Feeling Part of
Personality

Emotions

CENTER OF WORSHIP
Specialization of Emotions

Body Moving Functions

Sexual Functions

TAN TIEN

Instinctive Functions
(Biological Control Center)

Trigrams, the Sixty-four Hexagrams, the Ten Thousand Things. All of this, no matter what it is, no matter how dense and material it may be, from the highest spiritual concept of a God, to the lowest material concept of the densest substance conceivable (like a dwarf star whose matter on earth weighs ten thousand pounds per cubic inch)—Qi is everything from T'ai Chi to that dwarf star. *Li* is the intermediary, that which lies between nothingness and the material universe. *Li* is the conception of the material universe. The primary *li* manifests on a level of reality far removed from the phenomenal world. Wu Chi is the ultimate Real, Qi is the phenomenal real—that which is made to appear by the interaction of waves of probability with sentient observers. *Li* is that which forms the "laws" that underlie the possible manifestation of the phenomenal world. Qi is not real because it passes in and out of existence. *Li,* which is all ideas that ever can be manifest, in itself is real. It is the principle of ideal consciousness that exists inherent in Wu Chi. This *li* is expressed in the teachings of the Fourth Way as the Eternal Unchanging, the being state that lies between the unmanifest Absolute and the World of Three, the T'ai Chi.

2

Practical Examples of Li and Qi

THE CONCEPT OF *LI* PRECEDING QI can be illustrated with examples from everyday life. Basically, we can express the fundamental meaning of "*li* precedes Qi" by the proposition "Idea precedes manifest reality."

An architect conceives of a building. It may be the result of many things, including temperament, education, experience, employer requirements—but first the notion exists. If the notion did not exist, there would never be any building. Buildings do not happen by themselves, but rather they happen because somebody finds the idea in his head to build one. He sees it; then he draws, he writes, he makes plans. But the idea already exists in his head. That's why he's an architect, because buildings pop into his head, structures appear to him in his mind's eye. Then he places them on paper. Then someone builds them and they have substantial existence. Without the idea of the building, there could never be one.

Without the gene, the structure, the idea of a living form, there would never be a living form. Compared to men, genes are *li*. They have much less material reality. (Yin and Yang—you must always remember to make everything relative.) Compared to a man, which is a substantial reality, a gene is only the idea of a man. Yet if we can act on that idea in a certain way, and we can, through radiation and so on, change it, then the resultant being is changed. This potential to change what is manifest by changing the fundamental idea that proceeds it further demonstrates the reality of *li* precedes Qi.

People began to believe that the war in Vietnam was immoral and therefore must stop. So they protested, they complained, they sang, and they marched. This stimulated other activities. Organizations came into existence, they distributed petitions, they organized marches. Political figures became involved in the conflict, and the world divided into "hawks" and "doves." Eventually the war ended, and there is now a kind of peace. That happened because somebody got the idea, the notion, that things ought not be as they were, that something ought to change. Notion, *li,* precedes everything.

Some kind of conception of movement precedes movement. There is no such thing as moving without a preconception of moving. When there appears to be no preconception, it is called a reflex. But reflexes are already conceived in the nature of the mechanism; built into the machine, like the notion of "touch-hot-pull-back." It is not in the form of words, but it is a characteristic of life form. Part of the defining qualities, the preconception, the *li* of life, is that living things respond to irritation.

Can we speak of the cosmic man? Vishnu is the cosmic man of the Hindus, the World Soul. Adam Kadman is the World Soul of the Kabbalist. Because there is a cosmic man, which is existent in the Ideal World of Plato, men manifest certain ways, more or less in keeping with that cosmic man, and always as a reflection of that higher idea. Sometimes it's a good reflection, sometimes it's a poor reflection, but it is a reflection nonetheless.

One thing we must see is that *li* is in a different place. Our present day place is time bound; the other place is timeless. Ideal, *li,* is beyond time, and time itself is the result of the *li* of ordered events. The material existence, however, takes time. The material existence is Qi. There we must reorganize the Yin and the Yang. The idea is Yang, the activating force, which gathers the passive Yin matter to create the manifestation. The idea exists, that idea must affect the Qi, the Qi must modify and reorganize.

It is conceivable to generate a universe that is entirely different. It would be conceivable, if we could get back to the primary *li,* to the primary notion or the primary principle. But since we find that rather difficult to do, we work within the Ten Thousand Things; therefore, we reorganize on a small scale, while the rest of the universe remains the same.

Idea comes first. You get the idea of having a skill long before you finally develop the skill. That is why, when you get the idea of something, if you do it wrong you become annoyed with yourself, because the experiential reality is not conforming to your *li.* That is when you begin to change it; after a while you are doing it properly, because you have let *li* guide Qi. Insofar as you do not take in the idea and you do not let the idea guide the manifestation, you never get it right.

Li is fundamental and also timeless. Once you have a basic *li,* it will become clearer and more detailed and more subtle as long as you attend to that *li* and manifest the necessary *ch'i* (will). In the development of a skill, as in T'ai Chi Chuan, your initial experience of *li* relative to the various postures will be like the first stages of a piece of sculpture, a crude, rough outline of the final position. Eventually you are able to see that your position is not consistent with principle and does not look like that of your teacher. Then you are able to evolve a deeper *li,* which more closely approximates the ideal posture. Eventually you accomplish the new *li,* and an even deeper *li* can be formed. The idea is immediate. As long as you hold that idea, which is timeless, then you will slowly move into the proper position and begin to perfect it.

When it is said in T'ai Chi Chuan that *the mind moves the energy and the energy moves the body,* we are really saying that when you have adhered to the principle fully, and you direct your attention consistently, you will become independent of external forces and everything will be different in your experience of T'ai Chi and Qi. This change is a result of properly directed attention. By looking at the principle while carefully observing the degree of adherence to it, the manifestation becomes more and more consistent with it. You don't have to do anything, although it may appear as though you are. All you are doing is holding the principle and seeing the conformity or lack of conformity of the Qi to the *li.*

In T'ai Chi, after mastering the Form we take on a new *li* which is not only about the body but is also about the energy that underlies the physical body. Then that energy begins to be present and to be active. In one sense you might say that it's not true that a man has psychic centers, not true that a man has energy. He has nothing because he hasn't got the idea yet. But when he takes the idea and makes it substantial for himself, eventually it comes into existence. Jesus described that. He said that if you wish something, act as though you already have it, and it will be added onto you. That means if you want to be unselfish, you first discover that you are selfish. Then act as if you are unselfish. When a selfish person would really rather grab the doughnut from the table but does not, so that another may eat it, he's acting as if he's unselfish. If he makes that a constant effort, to act *as if,* he will eventually find that it is not effort and in fact he has become unselfish. That is how *li* begins to affect Qi.

Fundamental Ideas in the Body Centers

If a woman announces that she is planning to quit smoking, and does so with the lighting of almost every cigarette she smokes, it soon becomes obvious that there is really no *li;* nor can there be any directive force or *ch'i* (will) to act, since that would follow from the appropriate notion. I'll explain that in terms of psychic centers.[21] When a being is born, all of the notions that define what he is are in his genes, and the basic defining concepts of his life are the notions which are initially "in the belly." As a person matures in his early years, he takes notions in from the world all the time. These notions go into neither his head nor his heart—they go into his belly. Children take things in through a non-intellectual apperception, learning with feeling and with the body, and this process rarely includes any ideation. When you tell children something, if they believe you, they believe you within themselves, as a material, substantial, physical organism. As a result, children grow up with a series of notions fixed in them in the first few years of life.

At the age of four or five, a child becomes cognizant that people smoke cigarettes. What that means is "being big." So you want to "be big." When you're big, you can do what big people do. One of the things that you become clearly aware of is that big people smoke cigarettes all the time, because as a kid you can't stand the smell. But you connect it with bigness, with maturity, with freedom, with the right of being an adult. So when you're free to do so, you start smoking cigarettes.

Later, after you have read about the link between lung cancer, heart disease, and cigarettes, you become disturbed. You decide to quit smoking cigarettes. But you have the idea of smoking in your belly, in the root of yourself in childhood. You have a developed picture of the man who's harried and lights a cigarette. So you do that—you are getting harried, so you light a cigarette. Or you have this picture of finishing a big meal, then taking a cup of coffee and a cigarette. So you do it. These are the pictures that you have. These are in your belly. This has nothing to do with some vague idea about the world. This is deeply rooted.

Newly Acquired Li

Now you take in the idea that you're not going to smoke. But you find yourself smoking. You don't understand why you can't quit, even though you want to. It is because you "want it" in your head. By the head is meant the thinking part of the personality and not the higher centers of the mind and above. But that is of no significance, because the root of yourself is deeper down in your belly. How do you stop smoking? By bringing the new idea "underneath" the old one. When that happens, the old idea dissolves because you have a deeper *li,* a deeper notion. A surface notion will never change a deeper notion. This is why some people can be "involved" in esoteric work for their whole lives and never really change, because the only new notions they have are in their head. Some people get a little better at it; they don't want to be mechanical men in their chests. Of course, since the chest center is the emotional part of the personality, it produces only sporadic efforts and is quickly satisfied. But that doesn't accomplish the goal, because in their bellies these people remain mechanical. They have all these notions that are mechanically happening. It cannot be otherwise. You have the notion that if somebody says something to you in the wrong tone of voice, you feel hurt. But you say you don't want to be like that. So what? What have you done to find out and root out the notion that you have in your belly? What have you replaced it with? Do you *wish* that it was different? Only in fantasy does wishing make it so, not in reality.

3

Application of the Principle of Li to T'ai Chi Chuan

*T*HIS IS JUST HOW IT WORKS in T'ai Chi Chuan. You begin T'ai Chi Chuan with the notion that you are already relaxed, as you are. But you are not relaxed by the standards of T'ai Chi Chuan. As you begin to understand what relaxation is and become conscious of the tensions in your body, concomitantly developing new notions about the potential of that body, then you can change yourself. But these notions have to be brought down into your belly. The first thing to do in the effort to convert ordinary T'ai Chi Chuan practice into fundamental T'ai Chi Kung is to try to change the center of gravity of one's being. Normally in life, the center that has the greatest weight in directing the activity and thought of the organism is either the head or the chest. This is not meant in the esoteric sense of a yogi who has consciousness centered in his head, or in the sense of a Bhakti, or a man of God, who is centered in love of God or centered in love of mankind. I mean that *as you are, the center of gravity of your being lies in your mechanical-emotional center.*

The Chest center, which includes the area from the solar plexus to a point several inches below the interclavicular notch (center of the collarbone), is the place where you are aware of yourself. This is where your emotions reside and this is where you spend your life, in your emotional center. Because the emotions are fragmented and uncooperative, your life is usually like a roller coaster in its emotional ups and downs. Many different ideas and values are brought into the emotional center as one moves through life. Although many of the adopted ideas and desires are held in the chest and expressed in the head, most of them have little force as they are only atop the mass for a short time before some event or memory triggers the emergence of a different emotion. Yet while all this activity is taking place and your mind is engaged in imaginary choosing and deciding and explaining, you are living from your belly, from the values born with you or impressed on your root center in early life. It is necessary first to recognize that much of the fundamental energy developed in the body is "lifted" out of the three lower centers in the belly and brought into the Chest center to feed emotions. This energy, which is essentially *wasted* by emotional expression, could be used to bring new *li* under the entrenched *li* in the belly. Subsequently it can be used for the development of the energy body. Therefore we begin to free ourselves from some of the ordinary emotional turmoil by postural modification and mental direction oriented toward dropping all possible energy from the chest into the belly. When you finally do become conscious *in* the three lower centers, you will also become conscious of your notions, of your *li.* When you really do that, you begin to have what is called "gut response" to more and more things. Through observation and analysis of the deeper and more substantial gut response to more and more things, you become much more aware of what your underlying values are, and thus you acquire a much deeper and often sobering understanding of what your manifest personality really is. You begin to discover how little your mental and emotional pictures conform to the reality of what you have become as a being manifest in the world. When you then try to change yourself from your belly, you change. That's why T'ai Chi Chuan focuses on the *tan tien* or belly, for it is the place from which real change can be made in your life and behavior. It is, therefore, the place from which the process of transformation, the focus of T'ai Chi Kung, begins.

Man's Tension as Psychic Armor

We start the process of T'ai Chi Kung by working on awareness and control of the physical mechanism. One of the most basic problems to be addressed in T'ai Chi Chuan is that of tension in connective tissue—in muscle, in tendons, in arterial walls—even in ligament and bone. These various levels of tension are addressed from the most external inward. We begin by dealing with the general idea of "being relaxed." Most people have the notion that they are indeed relaxed (unless they are the so-called class A personality, which appears to intentionally embrace stress), but that notion lies primarily in the head; it is expressed without any connection to emotional or physical states. It is not in the heart, as there is no desire to attain a state of relaxation; in fact, there is no awareness normally of the state of the body. Deep down in the emotional nature of man is an intrinsic sense of needing protection. Every animal has an intrinsic sense of being required to defend itself. Unlike natural creatures who defend against physical attacks from the world with naturally developed defensive means, modern man defends unconsciously against the real and imagined attacks from the world with the tension of his body and covering noise of his mind—with his psychic armor. It is, in fact, as natural for civilized man to defend as he does with his psychic armor as it is for creatures to defend with claw and tooth, for he defends against attacks which are not the simple food and territorially rooted violence of creatures, but rather the complex and subtle manipulations of obligations, responsibilities, images, etc. In a really healthy environment for an animal, like a jungle, where there are trees and caves and natural cycles, an animal relaxes in its "cave" and tenses in the jungle. Even a domestic cat finds itself a nice safe place, curls up or stretches out and puts its alertness into its senses, listening for danger or for food, while the rest of its body appears to go limp. Even the gazelle herd remains calm and relaxed in the presence of a well-fed lion. When the lion grows hungry and restless, the herd responds with tension and eventually flight.

Man no longer relates to the world that way. He is no longer threatened biologically by being attacked and eaten by bigger animals. As a result, his defense is against things that are not substantial. He is ready to defend himself with his body against verbal attack, against attitudes that are not pleasing to him, against circumstances that do not meet his requirements or comfort needs, and so on. He is constantly in a state of tension. He goes into his own bedroom and remains in a state of tension, defending himself against his own thoughts. He does not want to face certain kinds of feelings, thoughts, needs, ideas that exist in his presence, so he blocks them out through tension. Thus deep in his belly he is constantly requiring tension of himself, but in his head he thinks he is relaxed, or at least thinks that he wants to be relaxed.

How does he change? By becoming awake to the reality of what he is—by seeing the truth about himself. By seeing this truth, he becomes cognizant of the notions that lie in his belly. By doing that, he becomes capable of formulating other notions to replace the existent ones. Until he is conscious of the notions that are there, he does not know how or with what to replace them.

I want to remind you that the ideas presented here must be pondered. Unless you take these ideas and think about them, analyze them, evaluate them, they will never even become notions in your head. To make these ideas real and make them work consistently, you must take them first into your head and know them in words as *li*. Then you must take them into your heart and feel that you want this to be real for you as a *li*. Then you must apply them to the world and to yourself, and evaluate the results and implications of those results. Then finally you have to put them in your belly and replace those other *li*s which are there with the *li*s that are being given now. *If you look at the world in a new way, you will see a new world, and you will be a new part of that new world.*

Summary of the Developmental Process Leading to Teh

As man is in the world, he has no contact except by occasional accident with the higher parts of his true nature. What he calls his thoughts, including the notions "in his head," and what he calls his feelings, his convictions, even his beliefs and desires, are not real thoughts and emotions from the thinking and feeling centers. Rather they are mechanical functions produced by the interaction of the body with the world in normal animal fashion, in a creature with a mind that mechanically needs to believe that it is in fact controlling its destiny. In addition, the three lower centers—the moving, sex, and instinctive centers—are in fact real centers and their functions are the correct functions, although only the lowest functions are usually developed. T'ai Chi Chuan, as the first step in T'ai Chi Kung, is the process by which the energy, usually bound and wasted in the two "false" centers of the head and chest (the thinking and feeling parts of the personality), is brought into the real *tan tien* center and maintained there in increasing amounts. Energy thus conserved becomes the basis for a number of different activities, depending on the teachings and orientation of the practitioner. Those internal activities are all essentially moving toward connection of the *tan tien* to the real emotional and then the real thinking center. These last two are, as a unit, called the Mind. The process of connecting to these higher being centers involves the conservation and transformation of certain energies which are already present in man, but only in insignificant quantities—never enough naturally to utilize for accomplishing any of the goals of T'ai Chi Kung. However, by proper effort, we can conserve the energy usually wasted in emotion and eventually transform it until we become conscious in the mind, and then in the body of discrimination, and finally in the body of bliss. These bodies are not crude like the physical-being body. They are not limited to a certain "shape and size." They have an energetic non-spatial existence—an entirely different principle.

But the intellect and the emotions that we normally contact, that we normally deal with, are very superficial and are products of the personality and body-type propensities interacting with the world.[22] Realize that your thinking and your emotions are all related to your physical organism. They are both primitive. It's very rare to have thinking and emotions that are related to something more profound than your ordinary self. The average person in the world thinks of heaven and earth in the crude sense of reward and punishment, all of which is related to the body. Most human emotions lie in the body, even when they're intense. When a person thinks of dying, he becomes panicky because he cannot conceptualize existing without the material substance. *Yet emotions and intellect are not material substance and do not need material substances. So it is not necessary to "experience the body to be alive"; it is only necessary to "experience the body to be alive," to be alive in the body.*

As a start for the above meditation, imagine what it might be like if one could exist in a state of loving life, or producing ideas that always helped life, but from some vantage point outside life? Imagine being a spirit that has no corporeal existence but that acts as a force for the well-being of life. Insofar as that would be coherent and would last, it could be called a form of "being body." Such an entity is said to exist in the form of Ishwara, a special Purusha who stays between the world of man and the Absolute and reaches down to help all yogis who call on him. He is invoked by chanting his name, *aum.*[23]

Again, these ideas must be pondered; they must be intellectually grasped, physically experienced, and emotionally charged. This process begins with the serious and directed effort to develop skill in the T'ai Chi Chuan form. This is done through careful study and analysis of principle and its application in the Form, while developing the necessary strength and limberness and coordination to accomplish the control of energy.

PERFECTING THE BODY WITH T'AI CHI CHUAN

體操

PART TWO

4

Acquiring Control of Qi

*E*ASTERN ARTS, AND PARTICULARLY the martial arts, have often been poorly understood in the Western world. To this day, most people do not begin to value or approach the tremendous mind/body discipline required of the serious practitioner aspiring to reach the heights of physical and spiritual development. Most students of T'ai Chi Chuan never even begin to experience the uncanny control of Qi that occurs for the diligent few. Most people, in fact, even most students of martial arts with whom I have spoken, watch the fantastic Chinese "Kung Fu" movies that are proliferating (with greater and greater depiction of skill and accuracy of detail, based on traditional inner and outer schools of the martial arts), and they believe that the skills demonstrated are either highly exaggerated or completely mythical.

Since 1979, we have held semi-annual health fairs at the Wholistic Health Center and Institute for Self-Development in Manhasset, New York. The fair has always included demonstrations and, wherever possible, some participation by the audience. One of the demonstrations always included is the ability to root. The first technique that we use for this demonstration is the Immovable Stance. When I studied a style of Karate called Moo Duk Kwan Tang Soo Do in Korea, the term Immovable Stance was used figuratively to describe any solid, stable stance. However, in T'ai Chi Chuan (and Aikido) the term is used literally. The practitioner stands in a Basic Box Stance with one arm raised as in Ward Off Right. A student (to avoid any participant injury) then pushes with both hands and as much body weight as possible against the upraised arm of the practitioner. One by one, other people add their weight and force until from five to twenty people are pushing and are unable to move the practitioner (Fig. 3). When I do the demonstration, I then walk forward and the people who are pushing fall over like a group of dominoes. We are sometimes challenged by those who see the demonstration and believe that it must be a trick. Even students of T'ai Chi and other inner schools have suggested that it was a trick or at least something that could be explained by the laws governing mechanics. They are obviously in error. In its simplest form the practitioner is channeling the pushing force through his body into the floor, overcoming the normal effort to resist. On a higher level, the energy is looped through the prac-

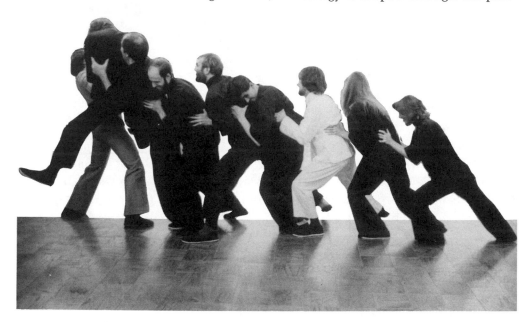

FIG. 3. Students pushing against the Immovable Stance

titioner's body and returned to act against its source, causing the participants to fall over.

In an effort to dispel the belief that we were doing tricks, a bias that exists in many Western observers whose limited understanding of science has led them to reject the invisible forces that man can control,[24] we began to also demonstrate the Unliftable Stance. The practitioner stands in a basic T'ai Chi posture with his arms as in the completion of Commence T'ai Chi

Chuan. The two largest and strongest volunteers we can find are asked to take a position on either side of the practitioner and to each get a good grip under the practitioner's armpit and as solid a stance as possible for maximum lifting leverage. The practitioner is easily lifted and usually makes it very easy for the volunteers by raising his energy and making himself lighter than a body would normally be. He is put down and the volunteers are invited to lift again. At this point the practitioner roots and the volunteers find that the once-light body has become unaccountably heavy. The greater the effort they make, the heavier the practitioner seems to become. Often they will turn red with embarrassment as the practitioner squats into a deeper and deeper stance, causing the volunteers to fall to the ground (Fig. 4). They attest to the inconceivable, trying to explain what they felt with expressions like, "First you were so light for a guy your size, and then you suddenly weighed hundreds of pounds." This technique is, however, not often seen. Although many claim to be capable of this ability to connect Qi to the earth and become fixed, none of the T'ai Chi practitioners who have told me this is a basic skill have been willing to demonstrate it.

I was first introduced to this skill by my wife,[25] who had learned it as a child in Korea from her brother (along with many other energy skills). I have one advanced student who has attained a reasonable degree of control of Qi. In the photograph, Fig. 3, the force of all the people pushing lifts a student, who is against the "wall" of force created by the Qi of my senior student, so the student's feet are dangling in the air. Several of my students are now approaching this skill.

Many reasons exist for the general lack of development of this kind of energy-related skill. One of the reasons is the unwillingness of many people to experience the pain of proper muscle development, either in the aspect of strength or in the aspect of stretching and limbering, or both. Another is the lack of effort to accomplish some of the musculoskeletal realignments necessary for proper energy flow. In both cases it is often the lack of instruction and guidance that leads to this lack of accomplishment. If a student is not taught, he cannot be expected to learn. Learning by imitation is easy when the teacher is manipulating objects in the world, as in cooking or assembling a machine. It is not as easy, but still possible, in activities involving the teacher's complex body movement, as in ballroom dancing, or popular sports and recreational activities. It is impossible for the student to learn by imitation when the activities involve the teacher's (1) control of subtle muscles and internal organs (2) musculoskeletal realignments (3) energy manipulation or (4) any activities in which conceptual guidance of

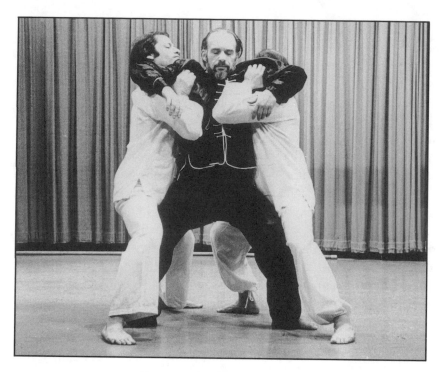

FIG. 4. The Unliftable Stance

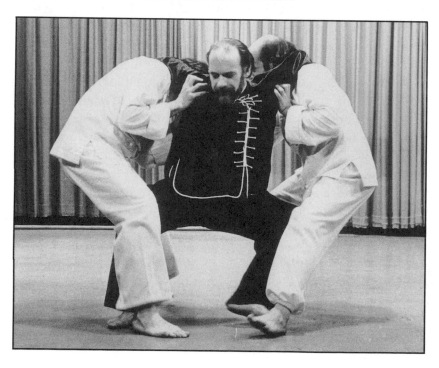

TAO AND T'AI CHI KUNG

the body is more important than exact body-part placement. Although serious instruction in T'ai Chi Chuan requires elucidation of these four activities, which cannot be learned by imitation, most students encounter the traditional non-verbal approach to teaching or "Watch, and do as I do." It's no wonder that we find a major problem in the unreasonably "cooperative" aspect of the average Push Hands practice. Instead of really competing and practicing the development of listening energy, yielding energy, rooting energy, and sticking energy, most students do what I have come to call the "Push Hands Dance," in which each partner cooperates in a pattern of movement that replaces yielding with retreating and pushing with following. This results in a sometimes rather graceful and T'ai Chi-like movement pattern which seems to satisfy many people, unless they are introduced to the real T'ai Chi Chuan practice. The student who is without the necessary philosophical background, not educated in the proper internal rotations of bones, unguided in the reeducation of musculoskeletal patterns, and who is not helped to visualize the internal pathways of Qi, can do no more than imitate the external appearance of his teacher's body. This cannot produce a practitioner of T'ai Chi Chuan.

The practice of T'ai Chi Chuan must be accompanied or preceded by specialized exercises designed to develop muscles that are generally not developed in most sport and fitness activities. These exercises involve the strengthening of muscles that are generally neglected, as, for example, the muscle on the front of the leg beside the shin bone and the muscles around the ankle. Together these muscles are responsible for lifting the foot and maintaining it in the proper position for the accomplishment of the leg and hip rotation in the Basic Box Step. The muscles of the inner thigh are another important example. These should be the muscles used in lifting the body from the position of Snake Creeps Down, as one moves into Golden Cock Stands On One Leg. To my knowledge, these muscles are only trained directly in ballet, and sadly, I have never met a T'ai Chi Chuan student who remembers having been told to use those muscles. The most important example, from the standpoint of Taoist Yoga, are the muscles of the back and front of the neck. This area needs special attention because our modern culture seems to have spawned a strange tendency to jut the head forward, producing an unnatural spinal curvature which negatively affects the flow of energy up the back and over the head in the circulation of the two midline energy channels.[26] (This is discussed further in the section called "Postural Correction.") Although many of the skills in T'ai Chi Chuan, including rooting and yielding, can be accomplished without this correction, the aim of T'ai Chi Kung cannot be realized without the free flow of energy through the *du* and *ren* channels. The straightening of the neck is necessary for this to occur. Many other areas needing serious attention could be mentioned and are in fact covered in the text that follows. In sum, much serious work is necessary for the real development of the body in T'ai Chi Chuan, and only then can it truly be called the physical part of Taoist Yoga.

5

The Mind and the Balance of the Body

THE T'AI CHI CHUAN FORM is based on the principle of the T'ai Chi which is circular continuity, as in channeling and returning, and on Yin/Yang duality as manifest in heavy and light, substantial and insubstantial, rooting and yielding, etc. It is concerned with the integration of psychic centers through physical alignment; opening of the *tan tien* and activation of movement from that center; rooting (connecting the *pranamaya kosha*—the energy body—to the Qi of the earth) through development of the legs and concommitant relaxation leading to sinking of Qi to the *tan tien* and, through the point Bubbling Springs,[27] into the earth itself. This rather obscure idea is expressed in a set of little-known writings called the T'ai Chi Chuan Classics, which are works of extreme brevity and subtle symbolism written sometime in eighteenth-century China. Normally this is the place where one quotes the Classics; the tendency is then to say something sagacious and leave the interpretation to the reader. This practice is both an attempt to carry over the flavor of the ancient texts into the present texts, as well as a method for the obscuring of ignorance. I am departing from that convention here to express the principles as I understand them after forty-one years of study and training in body development and combative arts, with energy development and control as the primary goal of that training.

Many practitioners of T'ai Chi Chuan misjudge these traditional expressions of the masters, in their so brief and poetic written teachings. They do not understand that vigorous and disciplined training of the body is necessary to produce sufficient strength in the legs, hips, waist, and back to maintain the correct alignment of the spine and other osseous structures while in motion. This alignment is often described in the T'ai Chi Chuan Classics by the phrase, "as if you were suspended from above by the crown of the head." I have often heard students claim "yes, that's how I feel." Yet these teachings come from a time when things were written as mnemonic devices, to help recall oral teachings. If students simply develop the image of this idea, in conjunction with so many others like it in the Classics, the straight neck and tucked chin and straight spine immediately develop. But so many American students of the martial arts do not bother to go beyond the surface of what is said. To compound the situation, they are often pandered to by an ever-changing panorama of masters from India, China, Japan, and the U.S. Marine Corps! (This in not a comprehensive list.)

There are teachers, for example, who travel throughout the United States teaching a technique called the Microcosmic Orbit in a one weekend seminar. They do not, however, teach the long, slow path of self-analysis and physical and mental self-discipline that leads to the ability to sit correctly in meditation. This means having the body properly aligned, with the eyes fixed on the tip of the nose but looking inward at the light manifest in the cavity of the spirit—with heart and mind empty of thought and feeling. Yet this is the pre-requisite for attaining the goal of the Microcosmic Orbit.

Simple songs, key words and phrases, a tradition of secretiveness, changes of meaning, of assumptions, of presupposed knowledge—these fragments left by the venerable masters form the seeds of esoteric knowledge that grow quietly within the practitioner. What I give you here will, if acted upon seriously for three years, bring you to a level of strength and skill in T'ai Chi Chuan—and any other martial art of which I know—beyond your expectations, and very real. It will then be time for you to feel and think your way beyond, for conscious evolution of the body must be done from within.

We will look briefly at two of the T'ai Chi Chuan Classics. I will make some comments on the meanings and then add, with comment, a few paraphrases of traditional "principles."

The T'ai Chi Chuan Treatise by Wang Shung Yueh begins:

> *T'ai Chi, the supreme ultimate, evolving from Wu Chi, the*
> *ultimateless, is the origin of movement and quietude, and the mother*

of Yin and Yang. In movement, the two act independently, and in quietude, they fuse into unity.

The first line should be a familiar summary of the Taoist description of creation. The next sentence could be interpreted to indicate the smooth transition between the Wu Chi and the T'ai Chi, which should be emulated in the art of T'ai Chi Chuan. The "two" may also refer to Yin and Yang, for at rest they indeed fuse, but in motion they must always be distinguished. This is mentioned in a number of places (see below) and discussed more fully on page 50.

There should be no excess, and no insufficiency.

Taoist writings on T'ai Chi Chuan put great emphasis on the concept of "no excess and no insufficiency." The concept is similar to the famous middle path of Buddhism—an effort to maintain balance, to maintain the center. This does not mean to keep the physical weight evenly balanced on the feet. In fact, that position, called "central equilibrium," should be avoided; it is not a good place from which to move, since it implies the point of T'ai Chi, or balance of Yin and Yang. This state, without excess or insufficiency, must exist on the emotional, intellectual, and spiritual planes. It should exist on the physical plane in passive meditation, but not in the dynamic and martial art of T'ai Chi Chuan. Here the body must always be clearly separated into Yin and Yang sides so that movement is never forced from the state of total, stable balance, but rather it is the result of a continuity of ever-changing or dynamic balance.

In spite of the myriad changing techniques, the principle remains the same.

Many kinds of movements in T'ai Chi Chuan encompass a variety of martial art techniques, as well as skills in energy activation and control. There are short forms and long forms, sword forms and broadsword forms, several staff and stick forms, as well as two-man forms, and various pushing hands styles and free sparing, et al. Yet the underlying principles that define the postural alignment, the mental set, the energy manipulation, and the heirarchy of movement, never change. All the styles and techniques of T'ai Chi Chuan are based on the fundamental principles, which are apparent in the movements if they are done correctly. Apparent, of course, only to those who are aware of the principles and understand their application.

> *Through diligent practice, one can gradually comprehend intrinsic*
> *energy and, from this, advance to the stage of spiritual enlightenment.*

To be effective, the very process of practicing requires several important things. First is control of attention, an effort to constantly return the mind to the subject at hand. Second is quieting the emotional nature. Last is relaxing your body. To relax your body, you must find out how to calm some of your emotional states. Unless you relax, you really can't do the exercise. The process of learning the Form is to some degree the process of calming the emotional nature. Thus with the diligent practice of aligning the body and sinking the Qi to the *tan tien* in the Form, the first of the three centers begins to function normally. If the practitioner continues in this effort and learns to straighten the neck as indicated (see page 110), the Qi can begin to flow freely and the practitioner will begin to sense its flow in the midline channels. With continual practice, the Qi will flow freely through the deeper orbit—down the front, up the back, and over the head—without the dangerous side-effects that can accompany Kundalini Yoga practice. If this process continues until it becomes "natural" and occurs without the practitioner's direction, it produces the biological equivalent of the harmonized energetic state of higher being, which will reverberate in the emotional and the intellectual center of the lower man. Under this influence, the intellectual and emotional components can be developed properly, and the practitioner will indeed reach the point of "seeing the mystery" in his lifetime. Then comes the alignment instruction.

> *The head top should be empty, alert, and straight.*

The state in which the brain produces alpha waves, often referred to as a state of relaxed non-specific attention, is the state of empty-headed alertness, valued in the Western world as a result of modern studies in biofeedback. No thoughts should be moving randomly through the head, as in the common trivia mechanism that occurs in most people under conditions where there is little or no requirement of attention. Thus the practitioner is not allowing any particular thing to control his attention, yet he is cognizant of the total reality surrounding him. His nonverbal thoughts are only of the requirements of posture and the control of Qi. Beyond that he is empty. This is a requirement that takes patience to develop.

Qi should be sunk to the tan tien.

Sinking Qi to the *tan tien* is one of the most fundamental aspects of development in T'ai Chi. This practice is described in detail on page 113.

The body is held balanced, without leaning to any direction.

This is difficult but important. I find that people's hips are always uneven, thus they are always leaning slightly and always cocking one hip or the other. The deviation between the height or tilt of the hips is something that must be attended to carefully. The pelvis is usually tilted forward or back, in compensation for balance loss or in a distorted conception of *tan tien*. The pelvis must be plumb, straight, with no deviation of direction, which means that the pelvic area must always be aligned, that the whole lower area must always retain its perfect alignment, its perfect balance.

Another work by the same author, in which the main theme is continuity and connection,[28] begins "This is the theory transmitted by Master Chang San-feng of Wu Tang mountain, with the desire toward helping all able people in the world to attain longevity and rejuvenation. The technique and art are the least thing to be concerned with." And he continues,

In any action the entire body should be light, alert, and coordinated, like a string of pearls.

He speaks of the body here in several ways. First let's try to imagine how the body, expressing the image of a coordinated string of pearls, would act. Each pearl lies in perfect relationship to the pearl before it and the pearl after it. When the pearls are coordinated, they're matched by size, they're matched by color, they're matched by lustre, they're matched by shape — so that everything fits exactly in place. There is no extraneous pearl; there is no part that is thicker; there is no sudden brightness. The body must move this way. There's no part that sticks out; there is no part that is separated from the rest. Everything must fit in exact proportion to the part before it and the part after it. Some T'ai Chi Chuan practitioners cultivate a kind of mechanical stiffness and prominent joint bend. This does not facilitate the flow of Qi and would be better softened and rounded to generate a greater feeling and appearance of continuity.

For our second image, you must picture moving a string of pearls. You'll see that it always maintains a perfectly smooth curvature. There's no place where it quite bends. It curves in a perfectly symmetrical way. The whole thing moves very evenly.[29] In the relationship between parts during movement, the body should be like a string of pearls. You must keep pushing parts of the body down and back and into place, checking to see whether or not you're moving in a coordinated manner. The hips must be aligned at all times, never allowing one or the other to raise up while turning. The elbows must be kept in the proper relationship with the body at all times. Movement must always be coordinated by the hierarchy of activity from foot to leg to waist to torso to arms and hands. It's very important to do this. This is one of the fundamental principles.

The Qi, vital energy, should be actively excited; but the Shen, spirit, must remain calm internally.

Shen is the human soul.[30] *Shen* is the emotional part of man, higher than the instinctive animal centers and lower than the directed-thinking mind. It is far less efficient than the instinctive or mind centers and more far-reaching in its effects. To maintain a calm *shen* is not very different from "putting a fishnet over the plentifulness of the heart." This is one of the more important martial arts principles, which is expressed in numerous ways. Grand Master Hwang Kee of Moo Duk Kwan Tang Soo Do, states: "Do not be a product of your environment," do not become emotionally involved. One of the fundamental principles of any martial art is not to become emotionally involved in the situation. So that in actual experience, when a warrior stands before his enemy, he should be absolutely neutral to the enemy. He cannot feel anger or hate. If anything he can feel compassion, if he knows he's going to kill his enemy. This is a very important part of the Form. When you're doing the Form, you must practice it with an internal calm, and this means also that you must keep your mind focused at the place and at the time of doing the Form. It is practiced this way because of the nature of the movement, the proper movement. With the calm spirit there is the production of free energy flow. The calm spirit allows the free and proper flow of energy. It also allows the proper alignment of the body. As the emotional nature is brought into a calmer and calmer state, the body relaxes more and drops more naturally into a proper alignment. In other words, the movements are meaningless when the mind is not focused. Most people's minds are rarely where the person is, physically. Their bodies are in one place, their minds are in another place. You must keep yourself totally focused on the Form and allow no extraneous thought to enter your system. That doesn't mean you won't think. It means that you never give extraneous thoughts any attention, any credence, any significance. Whatever does come into your consciousness is immediately set aside for later. All thoughts are set aside, and the mind is constantly brought back to the direct, immediate movement that you are doing. When you do that, you're really concentrating on the development of the mind and the emotional center, not just on the technique of T'ai Chi Chuan. You are controlling your mind, you are practicing mind control. You are forcing the mind through directed attention to remain fixed. You are not letting it wander. You are controlling your emotions in that you're not permitting any emotional disturbance. You are maintaining a firm control over your emotional center, thereby conserving that emotional energy. So that in working properly on the Form, you work on the other aspects of yourself as well. Working on tranquility is good under any condition, especially working on inner calm. What difference does it make to the development of tranquility whether it is developed through a physical art or through isolation or through some other method?

Now, "the Qi must be actively excited, but the Shen must remain calm internally" is a very important idea. Qi, in some sense, is actively excited whenever a person is actively engaged. We understand that Qi, the energy, is directed by mind, or to put it another way, Qi must be directed by something. Qi is not self-directed. The energy is not by and of its own nature capable of choosing a path for discharge. It must be directed by something, and that is either the mind of the practitioner or the mind and Qi of the opponent.

One of the principles that underlies T'ai Chi Chuan, and also Aikido, is the principle that Qi is directed by the mind. In Aikido, it is stated that if you can control your mind, and thereby fully control your Qi, you can control the Qi and mind of another. One technique practiced in Aikido involves "offering" your wrist to your opponent so that he is tempted to attempt to throw you and reaches for your wrist. As he reaches for your wrist you retreat at exactly the speed at which he reaches, and therefore, he begins to follow your lead. Eventually he will make contact and try to grasp your wrist. By directing your mind to the continuity of your motion and by engaging your Qi and ignoring him, your Qi will remain directed and you will continue to move as if he had not contacted you. His mind is now engaged in following your movement and is beginning to fragment further as it cannot decide whether to release or pull. His Qi is undirected, so that your Qi begins to lead his Qi. He's not directing his own mind, so his mind begins to follow his Qi. His Qi is following your Qi, because nothing else is directing it. Suddenly he finds himself going the way you want him to go. You make almost no effort while he makes a tremendous effort to resist, which doesn't accomplish anything. Anybody can do it if they concentrate the mind and the Qi. Thus when a person can actively direct his Qi and maintain a calm mind, then his mind is centered and no one can take his Qi or his mind.

There are always three levels on which to function: the emotional level, the intellectual level, and the biological level. Very often a person's idea is: "I don't want to be pushed. I don't want to move." By taking this "I don't want to move" idea and investing it with emotion—caring about whether he fails or not—he excites lower emotional energy, or desire. This in turn affects the biological level and ties everything up, affecting the biological organism in such a way that its potential is not realized. It is possible for the biological organism to be fixed and not move. It becomes that way by uniting its energy with the earth. That is, it returns to the state of being one with the earth. The only way it can do that, however, is if it surrenders, if it returns itself to its most primitive state of surrender: the simple, perfect alignment of the bone structure, exactly the way it ought to be, linked up between heaven and earth, linked up to the energies, not feeling itself as an independent entity. To return to that state is only possible if there is no emotional investment. The moment there is emotional investment in the idea, this organism is changed. By surrendering the emotional investments, by disallowing the power of the emotional center to control decision-making, by making the emotional force neutral, it is possible for the biological organism to return to its natural state. Thus by setting free the intellectual direction of the organism, this idea, "I don't want to be moved," can be realized. But it's realized through creative indifference, through an absence of anything in the lower emotional center. This Qi, this biological linkup, is a lower level linkup; it is an instinctive linkup. It is natural for the organism to be in that state. This is not a higher development. *In part, the development of consciousness means returning some of the primitive aspects of the machine to itself, bringing it back to its own nature.* Again, there must be an emotional letting go. Yet while the lower emotional nature is suspended, there must be direction from higher centers so that action (or purposeful non-action) will occur. This direction should come from the Mind, particularly from the place in the mind where Will truly appears (see Chart 1, page 8). There might even be a real desire to accomplish something for the world, for the well-being of man. As long as there's no emotional investment in it directly for you, as long as there is that position of neutrality, it is possible.

Do not leave any place with defect, unevenness, or discontinuity and severance.

The word "severance" is the key. When you begin to experience the connections of energy in various movements of the Form, you can begin to understand the difference between connected and unconnected energy. This interpretation relates to a physical sense of the energy connections. In every move of the Form, there is the possibility of discontinuity or continuity, of severance or joining of every part of the body to every other. When you practice the Form, when you make a movement, you're supposed to be making these linkages within the body. We define external energy links, for example, between the left hand and foot while doing Single Whip. You have to feel that settling in so that it sits just right, it feels right. This is a very important part of the Form.

But there is also another level of interpretation possible. It can mean that you also remain psychologically centered, and act from that center. Since we are warned (see quote on page 45) that the technique and the art are the least thing to be concerned with, the psychological interpretation must be important.

Jesus said, "When thou goest to the altar, and thy brother has aught against thee, leave thy gift at the altar and go and be reconciled with thy brother. Then return to offer thy gift." (Matthew 5:23-24) I think this means the same thing, not only in the Form itself or in the continuity of the Form, but in general. In *shen,* you must reconcile all things. Also understand that this reconciliation does not always mean actually to go and be reconciled with another. It means that you in yourself must be reconciled, that you must resolve your own experience. Usually when you say that "your brother has aught against thee," it doesn't imply guilt; it implies an account against him. "He's holding something against me" implies that you are holding him as wrong and you must be reconciled. You must resolve your relationship to that.

Energy is rooted in the feet, stems in the legs, is commanded or directed by the waist, and functions through the fingers. Starting from the feet, leading through the legs, and up to the waist, all movements must be acted as [sic] an integral whole. In case one fails in mastering [this], his body will be in disorder and confusion. The only way to avoid the pitfall of disintegration is by adjusting one's legs and waist. The principle applies irrespective of all the directions, above or below, front or back, left or right.

This tells us several important things about the continuity as well as the functions of various body sections. The practitioner should always be aware of the body, starting with awareness of the feet and continuing through the leg, the waist, the shoulders, and the arms and hands. The waist (the *tan tien* and hips) is the source of motion, but that motion uses the leg as a fulcrum and the foot as the anchor of that fulcrum. The waist is the place that joins the hips and the torso, and therefore the rotation of the waist tends to maintain the alignment of the shoulders with the hips, unless something interferes with the rotation of the shoulders. Once the torso becomes activated, the force is transferred into the arms and hands for the final execution of the technique. In terms of energy, the source of Qi is ultimately in the union of the Qi of the practitioner with the Qi of the earth (see point 2, page 54). When this connection is established, all activity becomes rooted in the foot. As the force flows up from the ball of the foot through the leg, activates the waist, and passes the energy from the torso through the shoulder and arms and hands, the movement should feel continuous from foot to hand, without any force added at any joint. The *absence* of added force should be particularly noticeable at the shoulder and elbow, since these are the joints that are used most often as the fulcrum of movements by most practitioners of martial arts and sports. This is best seen in Pushing Hands practice when the superior practitioner takes the force of his opponent's push, brings it down to the earth and then back up through his own leg, waist, torso, shoulder, arm, and hand, virtually as one unit, while the opponent feels nothing of resistance, and nothing of force attacking him, yet finds himself apparently pushing himself away with the force of his own attack. This is technically called "yielding and return" and is one of the necessary skills to be developed by the advanced practitioner. Most people have difficulty grasping these principles without personal instruction.

All these movements are motivated by the mind or consciousness, not from the externality.

You never allow yourself to become reactive to a stimulus outside yourself.

If somebody attacks you, there's an action; you act, but you do not react. In Karate, we seek instinctive responses. For example, when someone attacks with a punch, your block should be complete before your conscious mind fully registers the event. This is seeking the level of response of an animal, which is far superior to that of ordinary man. In T'ai Chi we do not really concern ourselves with the fighting aspect of our art. First we are concerned with the proper activation of energy and its appropriate direction and intensity of flow. It is therefore necessary to always choose and guide the action of the Qi and the body. It is not necessary to think in words the event and your planned response. It is, however, necessary to encompass the catalyzing event in terms of forces and their directions. A serious practitioner knows this either from observation or from touch. Evaluation, analysis of choices, decision, and implementation are all accomplished easily if the practitioner is in the appropriate mental state of relaxed non-specific awareness, without random thoughts. Advanced practitioners can be apparently "moved away" by the first light force of the attack. Since the mind has set the body into perfect relaxed alignment, and it waits alertly without emotion or expectation, there is nothing external that could direct the movement in any way. Anything that touches it will cause it to move, but it's not a reaction. It's simply staying in its own state, independent of any external force, since nothing can be added to it and to resist is to acknowledge the external force. "All these movements are motivated by the mind, not from the externality."

In principle, it is of the utmost importance to distinguish between insubstantiality and substantiality. There is distinction in every place, and each place should be taken care of.

The idea of substantial and insubstantial[31] is closely related to the distribution of weight in the transitions of the Form. It refers, at least in the dynamic aspects of Form and Push Hands practice, usually to a state of transition parallel to the transfer of weight during movement. It does, however, refer to the "fullness of Qi" in any particular area and can also be equated with the degree of Yin and Yang in relative parts of the body, which is most easily seen in yielding and rooting. The difference between the response of a substantial area when attacked and an insubstantial area is dramatic. If, for example, one is attacked against the root directly, which is clearly the most substantial part (as someone pushing against the leg or lower adbomen), the attacking Qi will be either neutralized internally, producing in the attacker the sense of having run into a hard rubber mountain, or will be channeled and returned, causing the attacker to bounce away, or even fly away. An attack upon an insubstantial part, such as the shoulder or upper abdomen, generates immediate yielding and produces in the attacker the sense that he has attacked a mirage, or that the one he attacked seems to be unreachable. This must be studied in great detail once the experience of these opposite poles is obtained. The substantial/insubstantial balance will exist—although on a less dramatic level of polarity—between sides of the body, between legs, between arms, between hands; the hand on one side may not be insubstantial although that leg is insubstantial, as in Repulse Monkey. This must be studied as an advanced phase, preferably by the practitioner through his own analysis of the Form. To repeat, "all parts of the body must always be thought of as threaded together, not allowing the slightest severance."

This is so essential. Nothing can move without moving everything else. The whole thing becomes united. That's the key to proper technique. It's such an important idea. That's why as we do Qi Kung, as well as when we do T'ai Chi Chuan, there is a continuous effort to see how it is that the movements are really integrated, how there is nothing going on that is not absolutely necessary. No joint movements, in particular, should occur to produce results that can be accomplished by the rotation of the body. Every movement should be comprehended in terms of how it's all united, and how everything that happens is a result of turning from the waist and legs.

6

Some Important Principles of T'ai Chi Chuan

*I*N STUDYING T'AI CHI CHUAN it is imperative to understand the "why" and "how," so that the mind can be properly engaged in directing the body through activation of Qi. Although most of the principles that follow are not classic in form, they are in fact correct expressions of the ideas that the T'ai Chi Classics were teaching to their contemporary readers. There is a great deal of substance in what follows and serious thought and review of the Form should be done in light of these principles.

1. **The body should be as if suspended by the crown of the head.**

The crown or apex of the head is the point at which a line drawn from the apex of the ear meets the midline of the skull. When a body is suspended from that point the legs are hanging and not supporting the weight of the body. This completely transforms the relationship of body parts, since the normal compression of organs, muscles, and joints is suspended; the shape and weight of parts define their position instead of being defined by structural compression. Observation shows that the large mandible (jaw bone) makes the front of the skull much heavier than the back, and therefore the suspended skull tilts forward instead of backward as most humans hold it. This forward tilt causes the jaw to be lowered and moved in toward the interclavicular notch, and the neck to be stretched upward from the rear and therefore straightened. The spine is rather straight, with the pelvis hanging plumb. The lack of compression between the lower ribs and the pelvic bones, as well as the lack of compression between the spinal vertebrae, allows much greater range of motion and much more separation between the lower and upper torso at the waist, which is imperative in Push Hands. The weight and shape of the rib cage will cause the ribs to drop down and in on the front of the torso when suspended, shortening the distance between the sternum (breastbone) and the navel.

Most people stretch the front of the body by lifting the rib cage and arching the back. This reverses the natural position of the body (which is rarely seen past early childhood). In addition to the negative effects on the flow of Qi, this produces unnatural counterstretching of the stomach, often leading to varieties of stomach problems that, when severe, can be extremely debilitating.[32] The corrected posture produces the necessary alignment of the skeleton allowing free flow of Qi. Further implications of this concept are covered throughout the text, in conjunction with other concepts that they help to elucidate. To accomplish this most essential principle a great deal of development is needed. The necessary awareness of positioning and stretching of tight and foreshortened tendons, as well as the strengthening and retraining of muscles to relax or to hold certain bones in position which are not usually controlled by the correct muscles, is imperative to accomplish the proper posture. Many of the preparatory exercises are detailed in the sections that follow.

2. You must be rooted like a tree.

In Korea many years ago, my Tang Soo Do Master, Ahn Kyung Won, spoke to me and another American Karate student. I weighed about 180 pounds; my friend weighed less than 150, but he was taller than I. Mr. Ahn said to my friend, "You are a lightweight man. You must jump and fly like a bird and attack your opponent." Then he turned to me and said, "Sohn, you are a heavyweight man. You must be rooted like a tree, stand and wait for your opponent to attack." From that day forth I practiced rooting in the simple manner of trying to feel all my weight sinking into my legs and then into the floor. I would visualize a tree's taproot and sense my energy as taking that form relative to the earth. Twelve years later, in 1973, my T'ai Chi Master, Don Ahn, watched me perform Tang Soo Do Kata and on noting the root and the circularity (which I had developed on my own as a result of the analysis of the movements of Tang Soo and their aim, combined with my personal aim of energy conservation and transformation) exclaimed, "That is T'ai Chi, Bob." The idea implanted by my Karate Master has never been out of my mind. Years later one of my acupuncture teachers, Dr. James L. K. Gong, in New York's Chinatown, visited my karate dojang and decided to accept me as an advanced pupil; my studies with him shed new insight into the relationship between T'ai Chi and medicine. While teaching me the Poison Hand techniques,[33] he indicated, as an aside, that the point called Kidney 1 (Bubbling Springs) is the point through which the Qi of the practitioner is connected to the Qi of the earth. Until that time I had considered rooting to be through the heel and/or the whole bottom of the foot. I had made some progress, but at the point where I began to visualize and feel the point in more precise detail, my root improved rapidly and dramatically.

3. Yield to the slightest force, as a leaf in the wind.

One of the greatest difficulties that I have observed in the understanding of T'ai Chi, among even seasoned practitioners, is the application of the principle of yielding. Again and again as I teach Push Hands in classes I repeat, "You must neither resist nor retreat, you must simply maintain your physical integrity and allow the slightest force to move your body, but you must guide the direction of its movement with your mind." The problem lies in a tacit habit, similar to the issue discussed earlier related to relative motion. Just as we look to another body to judge motion or rest, we tend to relate root, yielding, etc. to the physical opponent of the moment. The opponent becomes too prominent in the practitioner's mind and most of the activities of the practitioner are bound in considerations of the opponent. In fact, the opponent should be almost an incidental factor. Rooting, yielding, returning, require very little attention to the opponent, but only to his effective force. Even listening and sticking energies can be easily accomplished with minimal attention to the opponent. This should be carefully considered. I make reference to the opponent as a physical body, with the mind and emotional elements. The Qi of the opponent is the only real interest of the practitioner. The resistance or retreat that is so often encountered in Push Hands is the result of the psychological response to the opponent and, no matter how subtle the retreat may be, as long as it is motivated by a psychological response of fight or flight, it defeats the real aim of T'ai Chi and disallows the possibility of fully understanding Qi.

When the postural integrity is properly maintained, the root is accomplished, and the practitioner is standing "normally," any force applied to the body should cause it to rotate on its root. (Unless, of course, the force is into the practitioner's root, from which it will be returned. This possibility is discussed below.) If force is applied and the practitioner does not move, he is either a rather advanced practitioner who can fully control the energy of his opponent once it contacts his body, or he has muscular tension and, following inevitably therefrom, no free flow of Qi and obviously an unstable root at best. Remember, large-rooted and unyielding trees go down in the gale long before the supple green plants, whose roots, far more shallow than that of the trees, are clearly more than compensated by unlimited yielding.

4. Create space as you yield, compress space as you push.

When you press, as during Push Hands, your opponent must feel that he has run out of space; when you yield, your opponent must feel as if you are far away, and he is falling into space. This can be accomplished only if the practitioner's rooting and yielding ability is developed, and his balance can be readily maintained. He must be able to hollow himself on withdrawal, in a manner similar to neutralizing between Rollback and Press. As he yields, he must maintain his opponent's distance by using his arm to buffer the opponent's pressing force and continue to hollow his body as part of the retreating movement, not simply shifting back on his legs while holding the body erect. Since the opponent's press will be against the torso, the hollowing will increase the apparent distance significantly. The more the practitioner yields, hollows, and sinks, the greater the space the opponent will perceive. On the other hand, when you press your opponent, you should extend into his space with your body, but not allow your root to follow the stretch of your upper torso. Here you must lower your body and maintain root while stretching the upper torso forward into the opponent, so that he feels that you have filled his space, and he has no place left to go. These dynamics must be carefully observed and corrected in slow practice for a long time.

5. It is unnecessary for the superior man to expend his energy against an opponent.

Once you have become efficient at yielding and rooting in the ordinary course of the many varieties of Push Hands operations, you should begin to seriously practice the control of Qi. You must learn to return your opponent's force and let his awkward strength work against him and throw him; you must learn to choose, without mental verbalization, what kind of response to activate and where the force will act. Most of the time your opponent will seem to employ awkward strength. Even if he has some degree of skill, the superior practitioner will experience the opponent as using awkward strength; that is, the strength of muscle tension and bone and weight leverage applications, instead of purely guiding Qi. The more aggressive an awkward-strength attack, the more tendency there is to respond with a more yang or hard style response, especially if the practitioner has trained previously in hard styles, as I highly recommend. First the practitioner must conceptualize the channeling of energy along certain pathways. For example, when your opponent applies force against your left shoulder, you must not allow any independent movement of the shoulder, but immediately conceptualize the force traveling instantly across your back to the opposite shoulder, down your arm, and into the opponent's body. You must hold this idea with your mind and maintain the proper alignment of the body at all times. If you feel that the force is acting on your shoulder, you must, intentionally and with the necessary muscle tone to maintain alignment, rotate the whole torso into the opponent's left shoulder with equal force. If you do this properly, you will eventually feel the result of proper alignment and conceptualization.

Once this control is established sufficiently to produce a sensation in the opponent of pushing himself away with a force equal to the force he is applying, the next skill should be attempted. Here the practitioner allows the opponent's force, either awkward strength or Qi, to rotate his body on its axis. The remainder of the opponent's force is allowed to traverse the appropriate pathway always from the point of the opponent's attack, through the practitioner's body and back into the opponent, through the practitioners opposite arm, but only after the rotation has begun. This double action produces an explosive force that immediately causes a falling or flying away of the opponent, who reports being lifted up. With practice one can allow the opponent's Qi or awkward strength to pass down into the root and return, so that the opponent literally pushes himself away from what feels virtually like a brick wall.

6. Chen Man-ching said, "Invest in loss."

"Invest in loss" so that the awkward strength may pass away. The meaning is simple but tricky, and many people work without result because of a basic misunderstanding. It means not to make winning in the Push Hands exercise a goal at all. It does not mean to make losing a goal, however, as some do who retreat rather than yield. The latter produces the strange "Push Hands Dance" that allows students to move endlessly through a pretty pattern, fantasizing that they are growing in skill because they are not winning and usually fall back easily at the slightest aggression. It means to focus your attention on listening to your opponent's body, using your hands as antenna to "hear" the tensions that vibrate through the muscles as he attacks or moves, or prepares to attack or move. Try to set up the channels of return, to yield freely to attacks to your insubstantial side, to absorb and return attacks to your substantial, rooted side; to never resort to awkward strength but to wait patiently, sinking, correcting posture, listening, and practicing. One day your reward will come when, continuing to practice and refusing to use awkward strength, you are amazed to find that your opponent is suddenly the one who is losing, and yet you are doing nothing new to cause it. Be forewarned: excitement and self-praise will immediately bring you down. T'ai Chi Chuan is the foundation of T'ai Chi Kung. The ego and emotional excess are fundamental enemies of spiritual development.

7. The mind directs the Qi and the Qi directs the body.

Given this, the mind must be controlled and directed by the practitioner, and the attention must never be allowed to be drawn by any outside stimulus, or the Qi will follow the mind, and the value of the body moving in the Form will be no more than any calisthenic exercise at best.

The flow of Qi is dependent on a number of additional factors:

Opening of joints. The inability to properly control the points of attachment of the limbs, particularly at the groin and armpit/shoulder areas, is one of the factors that mitigates against many students ever accomplishing the control of Qi, even those who look as though they are doing things properly.

Strength in the hips and legs. The illusion that T'ai Chi Chuan requires little or no strength (which is true when, for example, the "dance" is used therapeutically with heart patients, etc.) has captured many who are unwilling to learn Karate and other martial arts, because of the strain and stress of those arts. Yet serious athletes have been amazed; one baseball All-Star for example, commented while studying T'ai Chi Chuan for about three months, "I thought I knew what it was to be in shape until I started to study T'ai Chi Chuan." A wide variety of muscles, some of which many people do not even realize exist, need development.

Sinking. Sufficient Qi must sink to the *tan tien* to provide impetus for the flow of energy through the channels.

Harmony of shen and po. The human soul (in the heart) and animal soul (in the lungs)—*shen* and *po* respectively—must be harmonized to guide the gross body to channel Qi properly.

Aspects of the first two points above are covered in the section on stretching and strengthening exercises which follows. Aspects of the last points are discussed mainly in the sections above.[34]

ACTIVATING
THE QI
IN
T'AI CHI
CHUAN

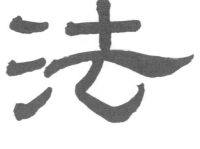
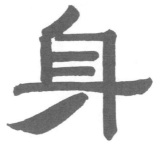

PART THREE

7

Benefits of Practicing the Form

THE T'AI CHI CHUAN FORM, as so many other goal-directed arts that have been adopted as popular pastimes in America, has lost much of its original purpose. In fact, so much so that to many students it seems like an end-in-itself—a solo "dance" that helps in general relaxation and may even be instrumental in the cure of some minor internal discomforts. There is limited and rather uninformed discussion about the place of T'ai Chi Chuan in spiritual development as part of Taoist Yoga. Some reports are occasionally seen on the reduced oxygen needs of the body in T'ai Chi and therefore its value in the rehabilitation of patients with cardiovascular problems. There is a great deal of writing and talk about the use of T'ai Chi Chuan for the development of Qi and its value as a quality martial art. Yet the ideas rarely manifest as practice in the T'ai Chi community but rather remain the subject of abstract, intellectual discussion. All of these qualities are actually true of T'ai Chi, either in its expressed purposes or in the subsidiary purposes that are intrinsic to the nature of the practice. The diversity of reasons for the practice of T'ai Chi point to one important fact: that the Form can be used with varying degrees of effort, and the results of these different levels are as diverse as the intensity of work effort that is exerted for the accomplishment of the Form. Although there is no question about the decrease in cardiovascular stress and increase in effective oxygen uptake in the practice of T'ai Chi Chuan by anyone with a reasonable degree of patience and attention, that level of accomplishment is not a primary aim of T'ai Chi. It is, in fact, one of the many secondary gains of serious intense practice, which include, but are not limited to, the following:

1. *Greater physical power* results from the increased flow of Qi through the muscles, increased strength in the legs and lower torso (the seat of real power as it is known to all serious athletes and martial artists) and decreased oxygen needs, which is a basic function of T'ai Chi Chuan.

2. *Greater physical endurance* results from the more effective use of oxygen and the retraining of the body to use muscles more efficiently by utilizing only those muscles necessary to accomplish any task.

3. *Greater control of emotional expression* results from the dropping of energy from the emotional center in the chest to the body center in the lower abdomen, thereby reducing the amount of energy available for emotional responses. This control enhances all the other gains.

4. *Greater control and greater stamina in sexual activity* results from an increased awareness of the pelvic area and from the increased energy available for sexual activity, as it is dropped from the emotional to the body center.

5. *Less need for sleep accompanied by deeper and more restful sleep* results from more efficient and appropriate energy use, decreased aerobic needs, and a general decrease in the disturbing emotions that so often interrupt sleep.

6. *Less need for oxygen and thus less cardiovascular strain* results from the very basic practice of relaxed and efficient movement. This explains why so many cardiovascular specialists have recommended T'ai Chi Chuan practice to their heart patients.

7. *Less need for food intake and less desire to eat* results from the general decrease in oxygen usage and therefore the decrease in fuel burned. As well, proper posture tends to produce a full feeling after small amounts of food are eaten.

8. *Less intense emotional requirements* result from the control of the emotional energy demanded by the posture and the type of movement involved in the Form.

9. *More calm and inner peace* results from points 2, 4, 5, and 8.

10. *More stamina and energy* result from all of the above.

Note that I have referred to these gains as secondary to the serious, intense practice of T'ai Chi. Some degree of these gains will be experienced beginning at levels of effort equal to regular calisthenic exercise; significantly greater gains will be experienced at levels of effort equal to a serious Karate practitioner. But to truly realize the ability to "deflect the force of a thousand pounds with that of four ounces," to be "rooted to the earth like a tree, unliftable and immovable by many men," and "to yield without being uprooted, as a green supple plant in a gale,"—to be able to "hear" your opponent's Qi,[35] to lead his Qi, to uproot him without expending force, to be the master of Qi, and therefore of yourself and all who contact you—for this, you must work very hard indeed.

Before beginning a detailed discussion of the adjunct exercises, I want to put T'ai Chi Chuan into a perspective relative to martial arts training traditions, which again will lay emphasis on the need for pre- and co-requisite exercise. In China there have been two traditional branches of the martial arts. These are then, of course, subdivided into the various real and mythical categories necessary to satisfy the Chinese scholarly need for order—an order that is not at all clear or comfortable for Western man.[36] The two great divisions are Kung Fu Wu Chia and Kung Fu Nei Chia. Roughly translated these are The Outer Schools of the Perfection of Martial Skills and The Inner Schools of the Perfection of Martial Skills. The external schools are based on the development of great physical strength, limberness, speed, stamina, and knowledge of techniques and the points of application of those techniques. There are schools that focus on various combination techniques and emphasize striking with the hands, feet, elbows, knees, and even with the head. Some schools focus on grappling or wrestling techniques, others focus on throws, chokes, and limb breaks; still others focus on grasping with preconditioned fingers on "acupuncture points," nerves and blood vessels. Finally there are schools that train in sophisticated analysis of season, time, and weather conditions for the application of specific small forces at very select "acupuncture points" for the accomplishment of specific injuries and/or body reactions, to include death at a future designated time. The inner schools, on the contrary, do not focus on any external physical delivery system nor do they teach any specifics about where or when to strike. Although one coming to the inner schools is usually trained extensively in the outer schools, the reason for the exclusion of these specific details lies more fundamentally in a different intent. The inner schools are concerned with the development of Qi and the proper method of controlling and channeling that Qi. In T'ai Chi, which is the only one of the three inner arts (T'ai Chi Chuan, Pa Kua Chang, Hsing I Chuan) that I really know, the concern is also with the control and guidance of your opponent's Qi.

With mastery of Qi, all skills become the same—it is the power of Qi that transforms everything and ensures that the practitioner accomplishes his goals, from martial arts to spiritual awakening. So what is T'ai Chi Chuan? It is in fact a training exercise, as are all forms (sets, *katas*) of both the inner and outer schools of the martial arts. It is designed to take the practitioner through a series of increasingly difficult movements which accentuate and develop certain specific conditions and abilities. The exercises for opening the channels at the groin are one of the clearest examples. This involves strengthening the legs and stretching the very tight tendons in the groin, where the leg movements have become extremely limited in modern civilized man. The preliminary movements of the Form require only a 45 degree rotation of the body while balanced on one leg, and less than a 90 degree angle of the groin while separating the legs, as in Ward-off Left. As the Form progresses, the movement increases. Carry Tiger Back to Mountain requires a 135 degree rotation and greater leg separation. In Fair Lady Works at Shuttles, we are required to make a 180 degree and finally a 270 degree body rotation and a full 180 degree separation at the groin. The increasing rotation requires increased balance and strength. The increasing angle at the groin requires increased balance and significantly increased stretch, for Westerners and modern Easterners, of the muscles and ligaments of the groin, the inner thigh and knee, and the ankle. The T'ai Chi form in itself cannot *produce* the necessary physical development, but for anyone who has the basic stretch and strength, the necessary physical development is *corrected* and *honed* in the proper practice of the Form. Grand Master Hwang Kee of Moo Duk Kwan Tang Soo Do (a major style of Korean Karate), in his original text describing his style, outlined forty-two forms, culminating with T'ai Chi Chuan. It is apparent, therefore, that there is an expectation of certain development before beginning the Internal Exercises of T'ai Chi Chuan, Hsing I Chuan, Pa Kua Chang, or for that matter, Qi Kung of any variety, and internal exercises such as the Microcosmic Orbit and Sexual Energy Control. I have found numerous exercises over the years that have been extremely beneficial in producing the stretch and strength required to execute the Form properly. These exercises begin the developmental process of kinesthetic awareness, muscle isolation, and muscle-function retraining.

Physical training for the development of the body includes exercises and movements for:

1. Strength of the body in relation to itself:
   Support of body weight on legs
   Support and control of the movement of arms and shoulders with the trapezius and latissimus dorsi (large back muscles)
   Support of the extension of either lower limb by the musculature of the opposite side of the body
2. Postural alignment involving muscle reeducation:
   Filling the lower *tan tien*
   Opening the anus and relaxing the perineum (area between the anus and the genitals)
   Aligning the bones, including:
   - straightening the neck,
   - drawing back and dropping the shoulders into their proper position,
   - dropping the ribs and stretching the back,
   - hollowing the upper abdomen by straightening the lower back,
   - making the pelvis plumb.
3. Muscle integration:
   Coordinating movement according to the hierarchy of muscle activity, resulting in the production of cumulative power
4. Muscle isolation:
   Making maximal use of filling and emptying
   Utilizing body movement and momentum to limit muscle activity
   Using only the necessary muscles for movement
5. Range of motion extension in certain joints
6. Control of weight and balance with *tan tien*
7. Movement analysis and integration

8

Adjunct Exercises

MOST OF THE SCHOOLS OF T'ai Chi Chuan that I have visited do not employ supplemental exercise, and the performance of their students — their lack of ability to root, yield, or comprehend energy — attests to a lack of development through exercise. Over the years, in trying to overcome my own limitations and then in trying to help my students overcome developmental limitations, I have adapted exercises from many areas — U.S. Army calisthenics, Hatha Yoga, high school wrestling, ballet, and other martial art forms. Finally I was forced to develop a number of specific exercises to produce proper strength, energy flow, muscle awareness, and limberness to accomplish the proper development of the T'ai Chi form and Push Hands. Some of these exercises are written here for the first time and are explained with reference to their purpose and to the possible major sites of "difficulty" or pain.

Most of the simple exercise and basic T'ai Chi self-massage techniques (described in other books on this subject) are used regularly throughout many of the T'ai Chi classes in this country and are concerned with the relaxing of certain joints and the stimulation of certain energy movements. I recommend their use, although they cannot have the same profound effects on unprepared bodies as they do on a body that has been properly trained, strengthened, and limbered. I have noted, in years of careful and consistent observation, that the exercises most effective in producing root and yielding to any degree were those that developed the necessary strength and stretch to allow the student to truly follow directions. It is not the student's fault that he cannot follow directions. Consider that he has no idea of what is required of his body by T'ai Chi Chuan. He is given some calisthenic warm-up, some joint limbering movements, some self-massage, and then told to drop all his weight onto his legs and to release the unnecessary tension in his upper body. He tries, and he does what is possible for his weak and tense muscles and ligaments to do. The result is far from the effort necessary to accomplish the traditional "three year minor achievement." Perhaps, with luck and persistence, he can obtain a "fifteen year minor achievement." Tension, poor range of motion, calcification—all elements that effect the range of movement of joints—will hinder the free flow of Qi through the limbs necessary for the accomplishment of the T'ai Chi form. Stretching exercises help overcome these basic difficulties. At all major joints there is an overlapping and criss-crossing of tendons and muscles; this configuration provides maximal structural support and allows for a variety of movements. Since Qi also flows through the muscles and tendons, there is a tendency for it to accumulate and stagnate within weak, tense, and toxic tissue. This type of Qi stagnation leads to arthritis and rheumatism, as well as neurological and even oncological disease. Chinese medicine sees excess Qi as accumulating and finally congealing into physical form as fatty lumps, then benign tumors, and finally malignant ones. The development and manipulation, or active rotation, of joints activates the Qi and returns the body to its natural state of energy flow. The indicated diseases are, of course, avoided. Many of the exercises are concerned with stretching, particularly in the inguinal or groin area. This focus is in response to the importance of that area, as the base of the bowl-shaped *tan tien*, as well as to the fact that the full weight of the upper body is manipulated from the groin in T'ai Chi Chuan movement. It should be noted that Qi flows more easily through well developed and relaxed muscles. It is also significant that the increase of blood flow to an area results in an increase of Qi in the area. In Chinese medicine it is stated that the Qi is the commander of the blood and blood is the ruler of the Qi; where one flows, the other follows.

We teach more exercises than can be effectively practiced at each class. Therefore I recommend that students pick out groups of exercises that will facilitate correction of specifically noted problem areas. One usually effective way to judge the value of an exercise is simple—if it hurts when you are trying to execute it properly, then it is a necessary exercise. I should remind the reader that the comments in this book should be taken with the same degree of seriousness and commitment as they are written. It is not suggested that a newcomer to serious exercise take the pain indicator simplistically to heart or he may damage that heart and many other things as well. I am speaking mainly to serious athletes, martial artists, exercise instructors, etc.—that is, to people who have reached the point where they understand the different types of pain that the body experiences and the specific indications of that pain. For newcomers to serious exercise or to the martial arts or to T'ai Chi Chuan, this book should be used in conjunction with someone who knows and can advise about the experiences that occur during intense exercise.

1. Karate Side Leg Stretch

This is a basic and important exercise that stretches the eternally difficult hamstrings and helps stretch the groin tendons in several directions. It is helpful in correcting some common postural errors that many people have developed from improperly distributed weight. Stretching the tendons in the groin and developing some additional strength in the thighs helps to realign the pelvis. This exercise stretches the tight ankle that cannot easily allow the heel on the ground. During this stretch, pain can be expected at the ankle, at the stretched knee, on the stretched hamstring, and sometimes where the thigh meets the buttock, as well as other places.

Stand with the legs double shoulder-width apart and the feet pointing out at a 45 degree angle. (Photo 1). Maintaining the proper back and shoulder alignments, shift the weight onto the left leg (Photo 2), bending the left knee and keeping the left foot flat on the floor. Straighten the right leg (Photo 3), and allow the toes of the right foot to point up toward the ceiling as you rotate the right leg outward, on the back of the right heel. Keep the back as straight as possible, leaning forward from the *hips* for balance. The hands should be placed on the floor between the legs to facilitate balance and stretch. Use the left arm to help stretch the groin by pushing back on the left knee and leg. Over time try to bring the legs into a straight line with the feet pointing 180 degrees apart, and the right thigh on or near the floor. Reverse left and right in the instructions for the opposite leg stretch.

Some people have a great deal of trouble with this stretch. If necessary, the heel of the suppporting foot may be lifted off the floor as the knee is bent when sitting over the suppporting leg (Photo 4). Over time the heel

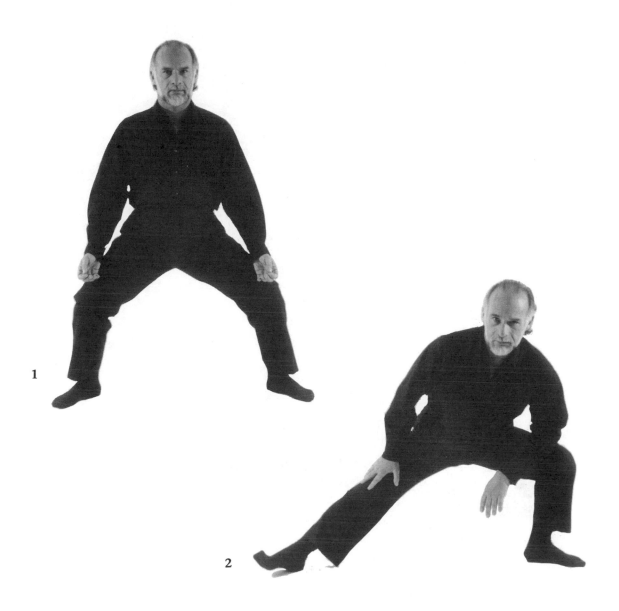

1

2

should be lowered to the floor for the correct stretch. This exercise stretches the hamstrings of the extended leg, the gluteal muscles of the posterior aspect of the hip joint of the same leg, as well as the adductor muscle group (muscles of the medial aspect of the thigh) of both the extended and bent leg. By gently pushing the knee of the bent leg over the toes as described above, the groin is forced open little by little, stretching the adductor muscle group[37] of the bent leg. This muscle group attaches the femur (thigh bone) to the pubic bone, thus forming the medial surface of the hip joint (the

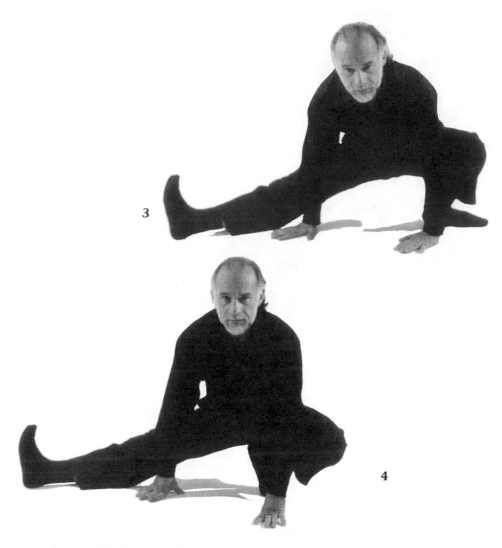

3

4

groin), which is generally very tight and often literally "closed" in most people. A closed groin not only decreases the circulation of blood and lymph into the lower limbs, but also prevents the Qi in the upperbody and *tan tien* from dropping and passing freely into the muscles and energy channels of the lower limbs and feet. Rooting is dependent upon being able to bring the Qi down to the soles of the feet and connecting the Qi of the practitioner with the Qi of the earth.

The muscles, tendons, and ligaments of the knee and ankle joints, including the heel and Achilles tendon of the bent leg, are also maximally stretched. The squatting position produces maximum flexion of the knee joint, as the femur and tibia are separated. This stretches the muscles of the anterior aspect of the knee joint,[38] which insert directly below the knee, as well as on its lateral and medial aspects. All the ligaments of the knee joint are brought into full flexion, thereby increasing the maximum range of joint motion. This exercise is imperative to properly accomplish the movement, Snake Creeps Down (Photo 5).

2. Seated Back-to-Wall Stretches

Sit on the floor with the base of the sacrum or top of the coccyx pushed back against a wall or other firm support (Photo 6); place the soles of the feet together. Allow the legs to drop completely to either side. Using the hands, draw the feet as close as possible to the body, without allowing the knees to be more than 12 inches from the floor. While holding the feet with the hands, become aware of the tension in the groin area, particularly the tightness of the tendons where the thigh meets the groin, and try to consciously relax the muscles in that area. At the same time, become aware

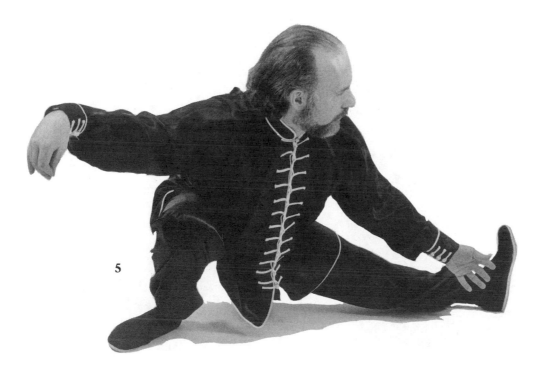

5

of the muscles in the buttock and thigh that can be used to pull the legs toward the floor. Consciously try to draw the knees toward the floor by pulling the leg down at the buttock-thigh connection. Keep the base of the sacrum against the wall all the time. After a few minutes, while maintaining the relaxation of the groin, bend forward from the hips trying to touch the lower abdomen to the feet (Photo 7). If the feet have not yet been pulled back close to the groin, try to touch the lower abdomen to the floor in front of the groin. It is extremely important that the bend of the body come from the hips at the acetabulum, the joint where the thigh bone (femur) rotates in the hip socket. It must not be from the waist, no less the chest and neck as some people do. There is no value in touching the head to the floor, for that at best stretches and rounds the back. If you hold your feet and try to press your belly and groin down and under with a straight or slightly arched back, you will feel an entirely different sensation from when you round your shoulders forward. You will feel the groin and its tension.

This exercise requires that a concentrated and bilateral focus be placed on the adductor muscle group. This focus should occur primarily as the knees are pulled toward the floor and secondarily as the body is bent forward from the hips. These efforts will produce three important effects: First, the direct stretching and opening of the groin. Second, the gluteal muscles of

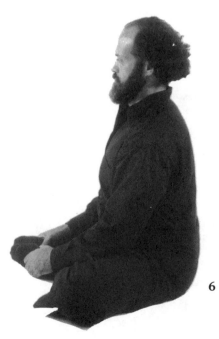

The wall is absent in Photographs 6 and 7 to give an unobstructed view of the alignment of the sacrum and coccyx. Make sure your sacrum stays flush against the wall during both these exercises.

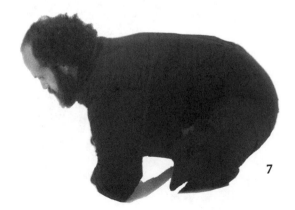

6

7

both buttocks (posterior hip joints) and the deep lateral rotator muscles of the hip joints are consciously isolated from the adductor muscles of the groin, which are then contracted and held. This helps to develop the essential kinesthetic skill of muscle isolation. The ability to isolate muscles is fundamental in accomplishing the T'ai Chi Chuan form. It enables the practical application of the T'ai Chi Chuan principle "no excess, no deficiency" which, in this case, implies using only those muscles necessary to maintain correct postural alignment and accomplish the desired T'ai Chi Chuan movement. Maintaining the knees in this position also strengthens the rotator and gluteal muscle groups. Third, an outward flare of the pelvic bones (ilia) takes place. The downward motion of the knees, with the back firmly supported by a wall, generates a subtle movement of the pelvic bones. This movement causes an opening of the anterior aspect of the sacroiliac joints, which is usually experienced by people as an immovable and generally painful area.

All three of the above benefits are maximized during the second aspect of this exercise, bending forward from the hips. Here the practitioner is required to "lock" or contract the muscles of the lumbar region to maintain the correct postural alignment and is concommitantly required to stretch these same muscles. This is an example of an "eccentric contraction," in which the muscles attempt to shorten (in this case the lumbar muscles) as they are lengthened during their contraction phase. Studies suggest that eccentric exercise offers a protective effect against later muscle fiber damage. Muscle training with eccentric exercises results in faster recovery time and less damage to muscle during subsequent exercise sessions. The same studies also point out that it takes a relatively short time to produce a rapid improvement in the ability of muscle to repair.[39]

This basic position, called Baddha Konasana in the practice of Hatha Yoga, is used for the healing of urinary tract disorders. Yogic texts state that as a result of practicing this exercise the pelvis, abdomen, and back are stimulated, strengthened, and receive a greater supply of blood. They also indicate that it keeps the bladder, prostate or ovaries, and kidneys healthy, as well as relieving sciatic pain and preventing hernia. The lumbar region of the back is a highly concentrated area of energy which is directly connected to the function of the bladder, kidneys, and the entire urogenital system. The opening and freeing of any blockage or restriction in the lumbar region will bring great health benefits, in addition to allowing the necessary energy flow into the *tan tien* for advanced T'ai Chi Chuan activities. Additional stretching occurs in the anterior and lateral aspects of the knees, as a direct result of dropping the knees to the floor while drawing the heels toward the groin. The ligaments and peroneal muscles and tendons of the lateral aspects of both ankles are also stretched as the soles of the feet are drawn together and inverted. This stretch helps in the lifting of the foot in T'ai Chi Chuan turns, which is an area that interferes with proper movement in many practitioners. The type of forward bending described above will increase the benefits of the following exercises.

3. Lymph Rub

Many years ago there was a T'ai Chi student[40] who had a great deal of trouble trying to stretch in a variation of the Back-to-Wall stretches above. He suggested this technique, which usually increases the stretch by several inches after it is done. It is based on the idea that the lymphatic system is often congested with a great deal of toxic matter and is incapable of absorbing more toxins. This results from insufficient muscular activity for proper drainage. The lymphatic system relies on muscular pressure from active bodies for stimulation, because it has neither the mechanical pump of the blood delivery system nor the chemical pumps of the neurological system. (This is one of the reasons exercise or physical therapy for patients who cannot exercise is essential. To lie still for long periods is to become auto-intoxicated.)

Place the left leg as if preparing to do the Lotus posture (Photo 15). Support the thumb of the opposite hand as shown in the drawing (Fig. 5). To locate the point indicated by the dot on the drawing, feel for a tight, nearly sharp protrusion. Using a small circular presssure with the thumb, rub slowly down the leg toward the knee. Support the thumb with the index finger as shown in the drawing, while following the pathway indicated. Pain will indicate that you are on the line. Do this two or three times with each leg and then repeat the Seated Back-to-Wall stretches. You should be pleasantly surprised by the increased distance of stretch, and more so by a feeling of increased elasticity at the joints in the groin.

4. The Plow

Several other Hatha Yoga exercises are useful for limbering the spine and for developing some degree of strength in various muscles. The Plow posture produces spinal limberness, develops muscular strength in the back, and stretches the hamstrings. Energy experiences will often occur while holding variations of this posture. The first variation is properly called a *mudra,* or posture that stimulates the circulation of Qi. Start the Plow by lying flat on

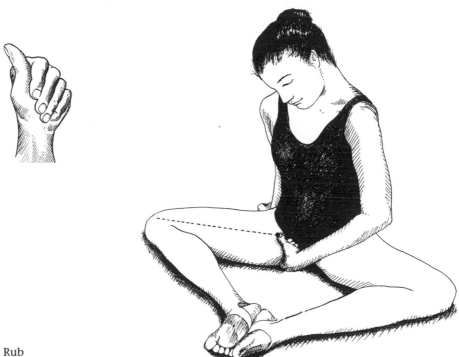

FIG. 5. The Lymph Rub

your back, palms up, and arms close to the body. The legs must be kept together, with the knees slightly bent. Keep the head on the floor, and, trying not to apply force with your hands unless absolutely necessary, slowly lift the legs together as in a leg raise (Photo 8). Continue lifting as the legs pass the 90 degree point and your body forms an acute angle. As the buttocks raise off the floor and your feet begin to drop behind your head, straighten the knees. Keep the legs straight and stretch the torso upward, trying to make contact between the chin and the chest. Eventually you will bring the toes to touch the floor behind the head (Photo 9) while the knees are held straight. When you are able to place the toes on the floor with your legs straight, you must work to straighten the back. You may use your hands to help by pushing against your back with the elbows pressed to the floor (Photo 10). Once the back is straight, you can begin the first variation which is the *mudra.* Stretch the arms back after the feet touch the floor, and, while pulling the toes toward the head (producing maximum dorsiflexion of the feet), place the feet, with legs straight, into the palms of the hands and cup the hands over the bottom of the feet (Photo 11). Maintain the straight back, straight legs, and straight arms, and wait. Shortly you will feel the flow of Qi around the circuit you have created. Once experienced, the value of this posture becomes clear.

The second variation increases the spinal stretch even further. After attaining the correct position of the basic Plow, bend the legs, bringing the knees to either side of the head.

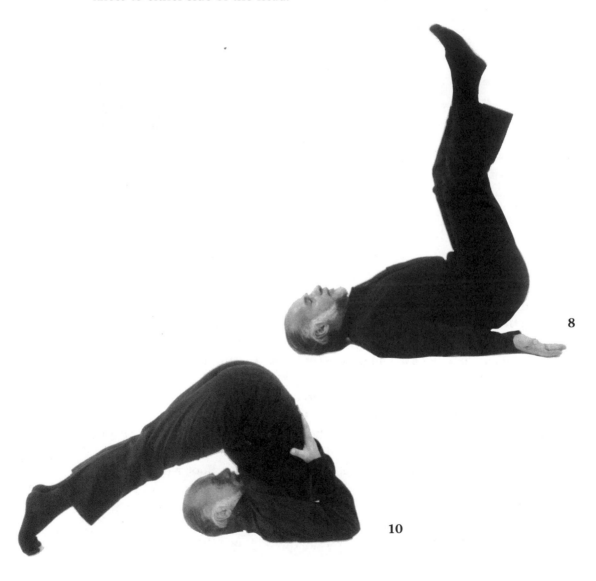

8

10

You may now reach back with your hands (Photo 12) and try to pull the knees gently down to touch the floor, next to the ears. The stretch will become evident when this is attempted. Whenever you get out of the Plow, first return to the basic position and then, using the hands only as necessary, lower the legs back to the starting position. Do not raise the back of the head from the floor when you are lowering the legs, or you may pull a tendon in the neck with very painful results.

Keep the knees bent slightly whenever moving them between the floor and the point where they make a 90 degree angle with the torso. This will avoid strain and injury to the muscles of the lower back. As the legs move slowly through this 90 degree arc, you strengthen the lower abdominal muscles.[41]

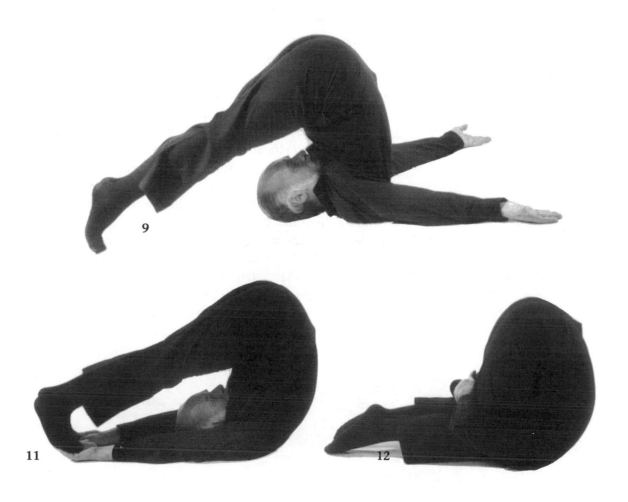

9

11   12

Strengthening the muscles that comprise part of the anterior wall of the physical counterpart of *tan tien,* as well as developing a deeper awareness of the specified muscles, helps in the ability to open the *tan tien.* When the toes touch the floor behind the head with the knees and back straight, the entire posterior aspect of the body is stretched, literally from head to toes. The muscles of the cervical and upper thoracic spine[42] undergo a considerable stretch. This is helpful in accomplishing the correct T'ai Chi Chuan neck position, which is described on page 110 in relation to energy circulation and T'ai Chi Kung. The area of maximum stretch occurs between the seventh cervical vertebrae and the first thoracic vertebrae (C7 and T1), a common site of energy and muscle congestion. This is the location of an acupuncture point that is the union of the six yang channels. Disturbance of the yang channels can create many digestive and urinary tract problems, as well as musculoskeletal problems (commonly found along the superficial pathways of the yang channels). Opening this area promotes the free flow of yang energy throughout the posterior aspects of the torso and four limbs. The Plow posture also stretches the paraspinal muscles and tendons of the middle and lower back regions;[43] the gluteal muscles of the buttocks; and the hamstrings.[44] Dorsiflexion of the ankles and extension of the toes stretch the calves[45] whose attachments to the heel bone form the Achille's tendon. This action further increases the pull on the hamstrings. Some straightening of the cervical and lumbar curves occurs during the Plow, so that the posterior joints of the spine (facets) and the posterior aspects of the spinal disc spaces are increased slightly.[46] This extension helps to free energy blockages that may exist along the spinal column as a result of tension and compression. It also stimulates blood flow and moves toxins by decompressing small blood and lymph vessels. The Plow also helps in straightening the back in the T'ai Chi posture; often slight calcification or excessive muscular rigidity related to poor posture, and many other disturbances, mitigate against a practitioner's straightening of the back. After some practice of this exercise, there is usually a clear increase in the ability to assume

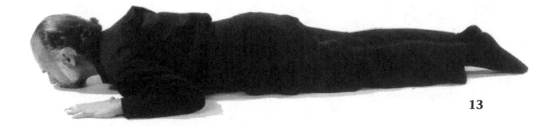

13

the correct posture. Bringing the knees to touch the floor next to the ears releases the stretch in the hamstrings and calves but increases the stretch on the entire spinal column, particularly the cervical spine.

The contraction of the throat, while the chin presses against the upper part of the sternum (breastbone), greatly increases the blood supply to the thyroid and parathyroid glands of the throat region. The inverted position, causing a change in the gravity of the body, allows the abdominal organs to fall freely in the opposite direction and helps to free constipated bowels, as well as to promote detoxification of the entire system. As the spine is stretched it receives a fresh blood supply, which generally helps to relieve stiff joints as in arthritis, lower back problems, and disorders of the urogenital system. Hatha Yoga practitioners consider Halasana, the Plow, to be a panacea for most common ailments.

5. The Cobra

Whenever the spine is stretched in one direction, it is wise to stretch it in the opposite direction as well. My favorite complement to the Plow is the Cobra, which produces virtually a perfect opposite stretch. Lie face down with the feet stretched flat on the floor (Photo 13). Place hands flat, with palms down and the thumbs touching the top of the shoulders. Do not use the arms or hands for support in the initial part of this exercise. Lift the head slowly, as if you were trying to reach toward the feet with the back of the head. When you cannot lift the head any further, begin to lift the chest, trying to feel the lifting of each vertebrae (Photo 14). It is important to be

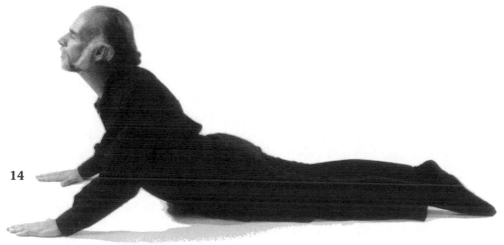

14

aware of the spine as you lift and to lift the head first, then the neck, upper back, mid-back, etc. As you feel the stretch in the uppermost part of the spine, you must lift the next lower vertebrae in order. When the head and part of the upper body are lifted, it may become necessary to use the arms and hands to support the weight of the upper body. Remember that you are to be more concerned with decreasing the diameter of the curve of the back than you are with how high you lift the body. Often one sees practitioners incorrectly lifting the groin from the floor. This is usually accompanied by a very large diameter back curve, but sometimes virtually no curve is apparent. The stretch of the spine is accomplished above the waist, so the navel is almost never required to leave the surface. (One variation of this exercise has the practitioner bend over backwards from the standing position until the hands touch the floor; he then tries to bring the hands and feet closer and closer together. This is called the Wheel.)

At the start of the Cobra, the shoulders are held back and down by activating the latissimus dorsi, the middle and lower trapezius, and the rhomboids. This creates an expansion in the chest region. All the muscles of the spine[47] are developed and strengthened by arching the upper, middle, and lower back, vertebrae by vertebrae. The tendency to tighten the buttocks and abdominal muscles, as the upper body is raised off the floor, must be overcome for maximum spinal stretch. These muscles must be kept relaxed throughout the exercise. This is training in muscle isolation.

The Cobra posture stretches the entire anterior surface of the body,[48] including all the major muscles and ligaments of the abdomen. Stretching the muscles of the lower abdomen will greatly assist a practitioner in the process of sinking and opening the *tan tien*. Some stretch also occurs to the quadriceps muscle group covering the anterior hip joint.

The effects of the Cobra posture on the spine are opposite those of the Plow. As the body is raised off the floor, the diameter of the entire back curve decreases, as a result of the increase in the cervical and lumbar curves and a reversal of the thoracic curve as the body moves into the final position of the exercise.[49]

In Hatha Yoga, the Sanskrit term for this exercise is Bhujangasana. It is known to help heal back and spinal injuries. It has also been known to help in replacing the spinal discs to their original position in cases of minor displacement. The full stretch of the abdominal muscles produced in the Cobra increases intra-abdominal pressure which helps tone the abdominal viscera. The stretch in the muscles, tendons, and ligaments of the spinal column brings a rich and invigorating supply of blood to the entire system.

The chest region is also stretched and expanded, helping to increase lung capacity and deep breathing, which is especially beneficial in respiratory problems.

6. Lotus Preparatory Stretches

The Lotus, one of the classic positions of Hatha Yoga, is, if properly approached, a fine base from which to practice several exercises. However, we have often seen people "tie" themselves into the Lotus posture—that is, force themselves into the posture with a calisthenic rather than a yogic approach. In this way, they are unable to use the Lotus position for its own value, let alone as the basis for further stretching and balancing exercises. Anyone who cannot comfortably—without strain, leaning, or body contortions—accomplish the Lotus and remain in it for several minutes without pain should practice the following exercise.

Sit on the floor, right leg bent inside the left (Photo 15), with the outer side of the legs as well as the thighs flat on the floor. The right leg is held parallel to the body. Grasp the left foot and place the ankle as far over the opposite thigh, and as close to the body as possible (Photo 16). Now, while

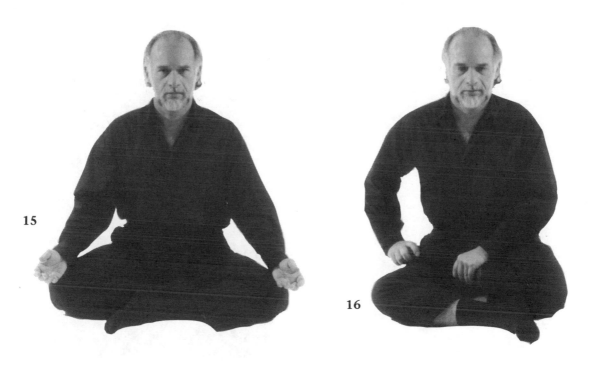

15

16

holding the body erect (not leaning toward the left knee), press the left knee carefully toward the floor. Try to keep the left foot on the right thigh; using the right hand, turn the left foot and leg so that the sole of the left foot faces upward, as you press the knee downward. Once the knee is able to stay on the floor without assistance, lean the body 180 degrees away from the left knee and once again use the left hand to press the knee down. Reverse left and right and stretch the opposite side as well. Once each leg can be placed comfortably in the described position, you are ready to assume the Lotus posture.

7. Lotus and Variations

The Lotus is accomplished by completing the first part of the exercise above (place the left foot on the right thigh at the highest, most lateral point) and place the right foot in the corresponding place on the left thigh (Photo 17). Sitting erect with the hands resting on the thighs or knees, you must try to relax into this position. If you want to get out of it fast, you probably have not practiced long enough with the preparatory exercises. Once you are comfortable in the Lotus, a number of variations can be practiced. First, lie

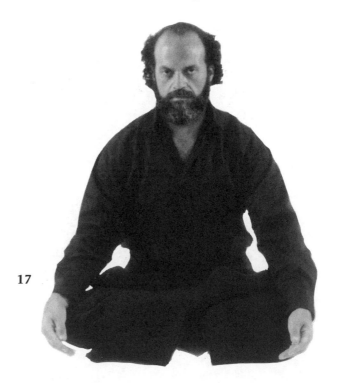

17

on your back allowing the legs, still in the Lotus, to point up at a 90 degree angle from the body (Photo 18). Place the hands under or next to the buttocks, and slowly and carefully begin lowering the legs to the floor (Photo 19). You will find that there are numerous protests from the tendons and ligaments at the hip joints. Be patient, careful, and sly, and you will eventually be able to lower and lift the legs as if you were doing leg raises, while the legs remain in Lotus. This exercise will go far to increase mobility at the hip joints. Again, starting from the basic Lotus pose, lean forward and place your hands on the floor in front of your legs. Walk the hands out and slowly raise your body onto your knees (Photo 20). Continue forward until you can lie face down on the floor (Photo 21); while keeping the hips down, lift the body onto the hands and arms. Keep pushing your lower abdomen toward the floor (Photo 22). This, too, helps considerably to free the joints at the hips and groin.

These and other variations of the Lotus position contract and work the abdominal muscles, as well as maximize the stretching and opening of the

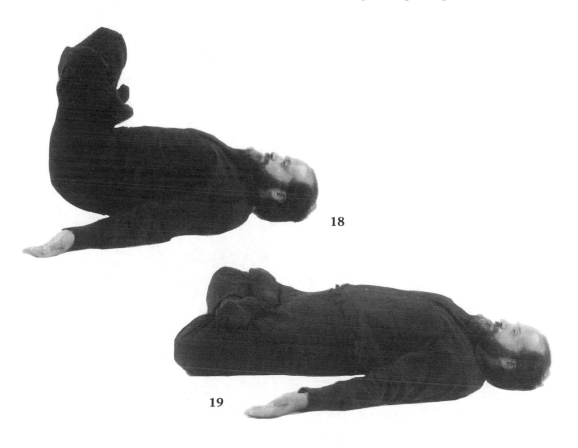

18

19

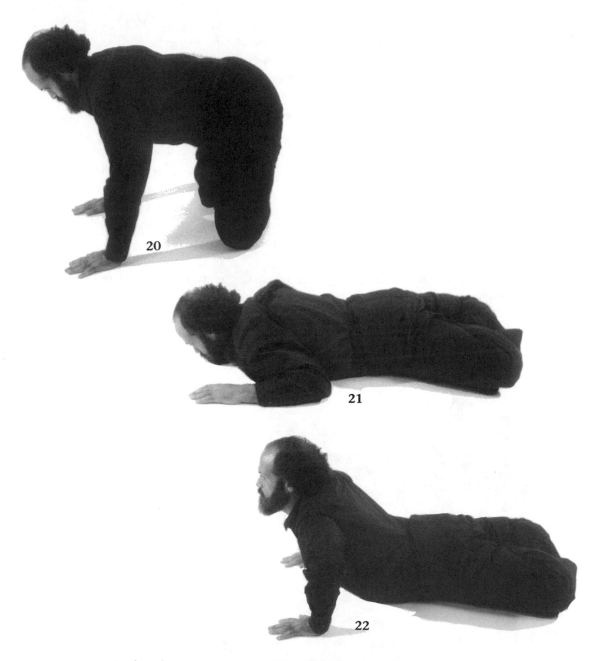

groin, hip, knee, and ankle joints. They also help to stretch and strengthen the lumbar and sacral regions of the back.

Drawing the foot and ankle to the opposite hip causes an abduction and lateral rotation of the hip joint, stretches the adductor muscle group and the sartorius muscle (the longest muscle in the body spanning both the hip and knee joints), and puts the knee in maximal flexion.[50] A major stretch takes place with the opening of the lateral aspect of the knee joint, as it is brought into this extreme position of flexion. The anterolateral aspect of the ankle joint is also opened, as the foot is plantar flexed and inverted. This stretches the muscles, tendons, and ligaments of the foot and ankle.[51]

Hatha Yoga practitioners maintain that the Lotus pose strengthens the pelvis, abdomen, and back while providing increased blood to those areas. The Lotus also serves to relieve joint stiffness, lower back problems, and to increase circulation in the lower body. Opening the lower body, as with the Lotus, will certainly have similar energetic effects as the other exercises mentioned which work to open the groin and hip joints and to promote the free flow of Qi. Physiologically, the greatest benefits are to the urogenital system.

8. Kneeling Position and Variation

Another important basic exercise is the kneeling position. Sit in the classical kneeling position (Photo 23), with knees together and the insides of the legs touching. Try to sit back onto the feet; do not lift your torso producing an arched back, but rather round the back slightly so that you sit as far back as possible. Once you have accomplished this you can lay back, at first supporting yourself from behind with your hands (Photo 24), and later your elbows (Photo 25). Finally lay flat on your back (Photo 26) with the back of your head on the floor. The stretch this pose provides the thighs will be quite apparent. To get out of the posture, simply reverse the procedure for getting into it: lift the torso with the thighs and abdomen, while first using the elbows then the hands to support the torso. Sometimes, because of weak abdominal and leg muscles, it is easier to assume this position than to get out of it. Lower back injuries similar to those incurred while doing sit-ups are a risk here. To avoid straining the lower back, use the thigh and abdominal muscles for all torso support, supplemented as necessary by the arms.

To develop great strength in the thighs, lift yourself up from the basic kneeling position until the torso and thighs are straight, and the legs and feet are still together on the floor. Now, *without* bending at the hip joint, lean back slowly. Most people will lean barely a few inches before they feel

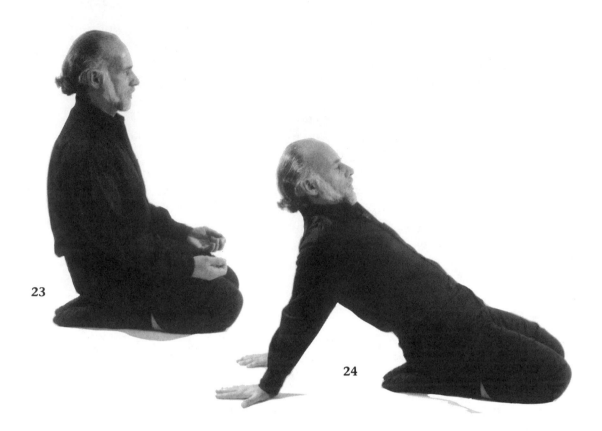

23

24

the extreme strain on the thigh muscles. Hold and return to the vertical position. Continue this exercise, and eventually, if you lay back and lift up again, you will be in possession of a kind of leg strength that is even beyond the basic requirements of T'ai Chi Chuan. By mastering this pose, every aspect of your martial arts, T'ai Chi, and anything else requiring strength, will be significantly improved.

For maximum stretch in one direction, try to sit between the feet. While in the kneeling position, separate the feet sufficiently to allow the buttocks to sit between them (Photo 27) but keep the knees together. Slowly lower the torso back between the feet. Be careful, the knees you might damage by forced efforts here will not be easily healed. You may then begin the same series of efforts to lay back as indicated above. You must be knowledgeable before you attempt this pose.

The kneeling position and its variations stretch and open the anterior aspects of the knee and ankle joints. In the basic kneeling position, the knees are in full flexion, producing a great stretch in the quadricep muscles

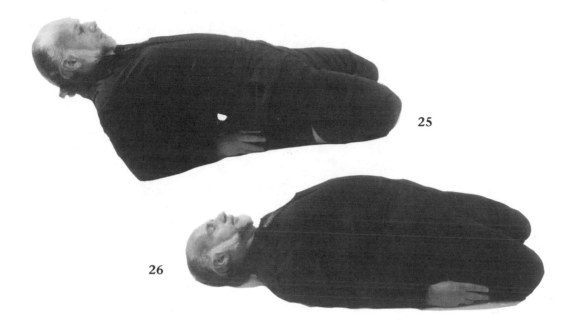

25

26

of the thighs and their tendons, which insert just below the knee joints.[52]

Relaxing the weight of the torso down onto both heels and feet increases plantar flexion of the ankle joints, as the dorsal surface of the feet are gradually splayed and compressed into the floor.[53] Allowing the back to round slightly produces a mild stretch and release throughout the entire posterior torso, primarily in the muscles of the lumbar and sacral regions.

Gradually lying back in the kneeling position extends the hips while the knees are flexed, producing a bi-directional pull along the thighs. This increases the stretch in the muscles of the hips, thighs, knees, and ankles and further opens them, allowing more freedom for Qi to flow in the specified areas.

Bringing the buttocks between the legs, while maintaining contact between the knees, increases both flexion of the knees and extension of the hips. At the same time a medial rotation of the thighs occurs, stretching the knee joint over its medial aspect.[54] Lying back in either variation of the kneeling position stretches the abdominal and pelvic regions including the abdominal organs.

In Hatha Yoga, the erect position is called Virasana and the lying back position is Supta Virasana. The texts on yoga state that the kneeling position helps relieve and cure rheumatic arthritic pains in the knees and ankles. With consistent practice this may correct flat feet. An essential pose for developing the health and flexibility of the knees, Virasana is also to be a remedy for varicose veins. Pain due to bone spurs on the heel will be relieved and the spurs themselves may disappear. The stretch in the abdominal and pelvic region promotes increased circulation and stimulation to the abdominal and genital organs, which, of course, not only helps cure diseases of that area but increases the flow of Qi which is essential for all the goals of T'ai Chi Chuan. It can also help to overcome certain sexual difficulties.

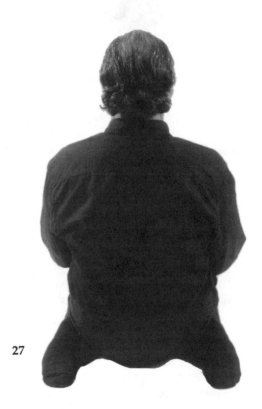

27

9. The Cross

This exercise strengthens the shoulder muscles, helps seat the shoulders properly, and slowly allows the practitioner to use the trapezius muscles as a whole to support the arms. This is part of the necessary skeletal realignment in which the humerus (the bone of the upper arm) slowly "settles" correctly into the shoulder socket. It also helps to flatten the scapulae (shoulder blades).[55]

Stand with feet shoulder-width apart and extend the arms directly out to the sides, parallel to the floor. Rotate the shoulders down and back and draw the scapulae down. Make sure that the elbows are pointing toward the floor. Relax the hands, but do not let them become claw-like (Photo 28). This exercise requires patience and forbearance. Wait and the shoulders will begin to hurt. As the shoulder girdle begins to ache, you can consciously attempt to transfer the sense of holding from the shoulders into the muscles of the upper back.

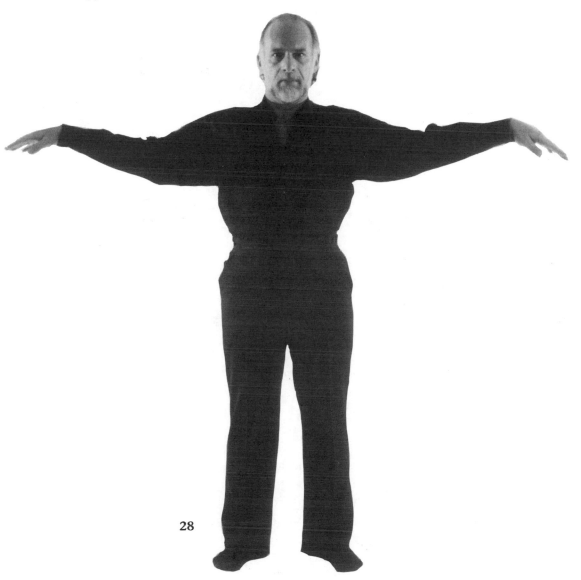

28

Try to feel the upper and middle back by alternately flexing and relaxing the upper back muscles, and imagine the upper and middle back muscles (particularly trapezius 1 and 2, the part above the level of the armpit) taking control. Try to picture the pathway that the muscles are forming along which the new control is occuring. As you feel some fatigue in the upper parts of the back muscles, try to feel and utilize the lower portions of the trapezius—first mid-back and finally down to the top of the lumbar spine. You are trying to retrain muscles to do what they should have been doing all along but have not. Persistence alone will bring results; this is not a simple calisthenic exercise, but an internal activity involved in part with nerve pathway retraining. It is very rare that anyone beginning this exercise can hold the arms up for a full five minutes. Persist in the internal attention and relaxation of the shoulder girdle and the results will be amazing.

10. Chinese Horse Stance Exercises

These exercises strengthen the muscles supporting the area that physically corresponds to the *tan tien*. They strengthen and stretch the muscles in the hips, buttocks, groin, and legs and thereby help in the development of awareness in the *tan tien* area.

Stand with the legs double shoulder-width apart, with the feet pointing out at about a 45 degree angle. Maintaining the proper back and shoulder alignment, bend the knees as much as possible, continuing to maintain a wide angle at the groin. When the body can be lowered so that the angle at the knee is close to 90 degrees (Photo 29), slowly drop the body forward, bending at the hips, maintaining the straight back and keeping the weight evenly distributed over the feet. When the body is able to maintain a fairly straight-backed wide-legged stance, with the thighs nearly parallel to the floor, reach between the thighs and behind the calves to grasp the ankles with the hands, left to left and right to right (Photo 30). Now shift the weight from leg to leg as far as possible (Photo 31) without compromising the back. The angles of the legs will change with the shifts but will always pass through the starting point described above as you shift from side to side. This exercise will produce strength in the legs, the back, the ankles, and the thighs. It will go far in stretching the groin muscles as well as the gluteus maximus where it joins the femur and the back of the leg. In some cases, it will start stretching the inner thigh muscles as well. If the back and neck can be maintained in a perfect T'ai Chi posture as you lean forward at

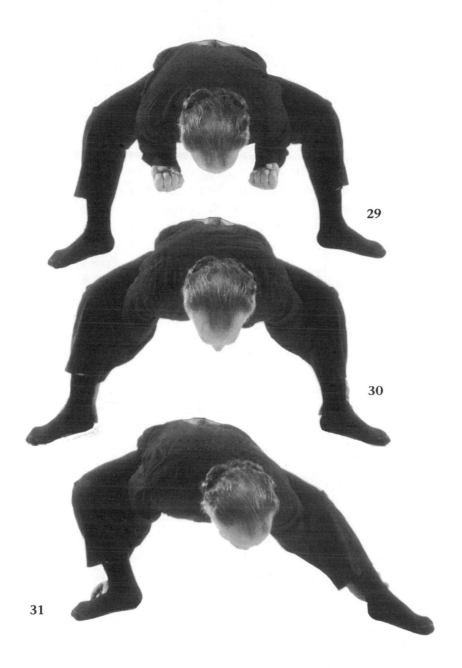

29

30

31

a 90 degree angle at the hip joint (*not* the waist), and if you can hold *tan tien* and can relax the body, you have attained the position of The Golden Turtle, which is one of the most important of Qi Kung exercises. This is much harder than you imagine. In my work with many professional athletes, it has often taken months for them to comprehend *straight* back—for

Activating the Qi in T'ai Chi Chuan

them to acquire the proper conscious awareness of the back muscles that enabled them to relax and stretch, and thereby straighten, the back.

Maintaining proper alignment is one of the key factors in accomplishing the Chinese Horse Stance. After the initial stance is taken, with the T'ai Chi posture maintained, you should relax and let the weight drop evenly into the legs. When this is done as described, the lower torso and legs should almost "lock" into position, creating a feeling of great stability. Eventually this stance will produce an awareness that the bone alignment is its own support, so that the muscles are all essentially relaxed. This awareness is important for success in the remainder of the exercise, as it allows proper muscle isolation. If you do not let go and relax into the alignment, you will contract most of the muscles of the lower torso and legs, to support the weight of the upper torso. This will result in unnecessary tensing of the gluteal and hamstring muscles, and the entire perineum area, including the anus and genitals. This alignment is analogous to the structure of an architecturally sound building—as tons of concrete and other building materials are added to the skeletal structure, the downward force of the weight of the building material is distributed evenly and passes freely down and through the metal structure into the foundation.

The Chinese Horse Stance greatly strengthens the quadricep muscles of the anterior thigh, which are primarily responsible for holding the lower extremities in the correctly aligned position. As the practitioner's hips and groin muscles (adductors) are stretched open, while trying to keep the knees aligned with the toes, the knees should bend deeper into the stance. This allows the gluteal muscles (glueteus minimus, medius, and maximus) and the tensor fascia latae to be more relaxed, while the wide angle of the groin is maintained. It also allows the adductor muscles of the medial thigh to move into their first level of stretch in this exercise. If the practitioner's hips and groin are not stretched open sufficiently, the gluteals and tensor fascia latae will contract to abduct the hip and thigh, in order to bring and hold the knees over the toes. Therefore, the Seated Back-to-Wall Stretches are necessary preparation for accomplishing the correct Chinese Horse Stance.

Bending the torso forward from the hip joints and not from the waist requires a controlled release of the torso by the gluteal and hamstring muscles, while the erector spinae and deeper muscles of the back, as well as the latissimus dorsi, rhomboids and trapezius muscles, maintain the correct T'ai Chi posture. The major stretch and opening occurs at the rotation point of the hip. The hamstrings[56] and the gluteals[57] are stretched as the rotation forward flexes the hip joint. These same muscles contract just enough to gradually raise the body back into the initial Chinese Horse Stance, while continuing to maintain the correct T'ai Chi posture. The quadricep muscles are strengthened from holding this position, while the adductor muscles of the groin are stretched even further by allowing the torso to rest between the thighs, forcing the knees to spread and stretch naturally.

This exercise produces a greater awareness of the *tan tien* and promotes increased circulation of blood and Qi to the lower abdomen and pelvic regions. Increased blood and energy to these regions brings great health benefits to the urogenital systems as well as increased sexual energy. This exercise also strengthens the back and helps in the relief of chronic lower back problems.

11. Bow and Arrow Exercise

This pose intensely stretches the muscles that attach the thighs to the buttocks. In addition it stretches groin, knee, and other leg muscles. It is possible to use it to strengthen the inner thigh, *if* the student makes the correct effort when getting up from the exercise. The latter makes possible the correct execution of Snake Creeps Down (Squatting Single Whip), which is generally accomplished by pushing with the back leg. (This is actually supposed to be accomplished by the adductors of the front leg.)

The name Bow and Arrow was given to this exercise by my students, probably because of the intense stretch that usually occurs at the buttock-thigh juncture of the bent leg. The exercise was devised by observing the difficulties students had making the transition from Ward-off Right to Roll Back. When the arms rotate and change position and the hips rotate to the right before the pull back from the right hip begins, I observed that most people are unable to maintain the proper hip and shoulder alignment; they twist at the shoulders into a poor semblance of the correct posture. This break of alignment is unacceptable to anyone wishing to develop Qi. I simply carried the rotation of the body further and extended the leg position, until I felt some stretching as I reached the floor. We have found the exercise is best practiced in the following manner.

Place the left knee on the floor with the left leg parallel to the body. Turn the right leg back so that it forms a 90-degree angle with the left leg. Try to push the hips forward evenly. This will be more difficult than you would expect. Hold for a few minutes (Photo 32). Lean forward and place the hands on the floor beyond the leg, being careful to keep the shoulders down and back, as in any T'ai Chi activity. Lift the hips evenly, while keeping the left knee and leg on the floor in the correct position. The left thigh, of course, will now angle down from the raised hip to the knee which is still on the floor. Push the right leg back until it is straight, parallel to the left thigh, with the right instep pressed on the floor. Do not let the right hip raise higher than the left (Photo 33). Once you are correctly in this position, try to relax and feel where the strains are occurring. Over time you should lower both hips to the floor and lie straight over the left thigh with your arms extended (Photo 34). Practice this on both sides by simply reversing the instructions.

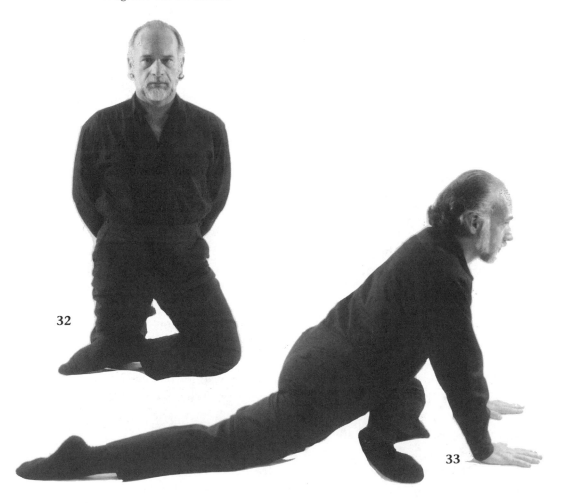

32

33

TAO AND T'AI CHI KUNG

In the starting position of the Bow and Arrow, the left thigh is laterally rotated at the hip, the left knee is flexed, and the left ankle is plantar flexed. The right leg is flexed at the knee and the right ankle is plantar flexed. This initial stretch, felt primarily at the left hip, is produced by trying to make the left hip even with the right by rotating and pushing the left hip forward. The left hip will tend to be pulled back and down due to the usual restrictions in the hips. Doing this pose correctly stretches the iliopsoas, the quadricep, and the sartorius muscles of the left hip and thigh. The same stretches occur on the right side when the instructions are reversed.

As the left hip is lowered to the floor, left hip flexion is gradually increased, intensifying the opening and stretch of the lateral and posterior aspects of the joint and its ligaments.[58] Extension at the right anterior hip joint is increased as the right leg is pushed straight back, parallel to the left thigh. This stretches the rectus femoris tendon, the quadricep muscles in general, and the iliopsoas muscle. The final position of the Bow and Arrow brings the ligaments, tendons, and muscles of the left thigh and hip into maximal stretch, opening the hip enormously.

Coming out of the Bow and Arrow properly requires isolation and contraction of the inner thigh or adductor muscles of the front leg. The laterally rotated position of the thigh, and the flexed position of the knee, help to isolate the contracted adductor muscles, which are used to lift oneself up and out of the exercise. The health benefits of this exercise are similar to the others that focus on opening the hips and lower body.

12. Karate Side-Kick Exercise

One of the difficulties that I have noted throughout the T'ai Chi world is the general weakness of the muscles involved in lifting the foot during the

34

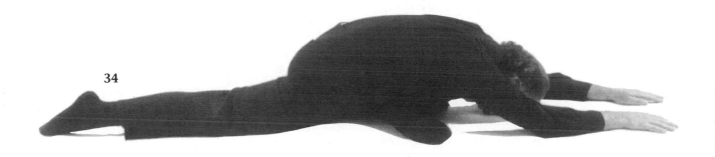

turn. Since this is an important factor in proper movement relative to the development of power, it is necessary for most practitioners to focus on development of the muscles at the ankle (particularly the medial ankle) and along the shin. The tibialis anterior muscle helps protect the rather prominent shinbone (tibia), which is often injured by blows in the marital arts as well as by strain-produced shinsplints. When the muscle is developed this does not occur.

Start the Karate Side-Kick by standing next to a wall, or other structure, using your hand for support. Lift the outside leg several inches off the ground, and pull the foot up into maximal flexion. Pull the toes up as well. Draw the foot in towards your midline. You should, if you are pulling hard in all of the three areas indicated, begin to feel strain on the shin and at the ankle. Place the foot on the floor, and adjust it until the blade (lateral edge) of the foot is the only part that touches the ground. The area of the blade near the outer ankle (external malleolus) and instep should touch the ground; the area near the toes may or may not touch. While holding the foot in the specified position, lift the leg and extend it sideways, (Photo 35) maintaining the foot position with maximum effort while keeping the knee locked in extension and the hips and pelvis tucked in.

When the leg is fully extended, look at the foot and adjust it if necessary. Withdraw the leg and, placing the foot on the ground, check the alignment again. Repeat ten times with each leg. Do this exercise often. It is very important, and its importance will become apparent after only two or three months.

While the dorsiflexion and inversion of the foot strengthens the muscles of the front of the leg, it also stretches the muscles that evert the foot on the lateral side of the leg. This stretch to the lateral ankle is maximized when the blade of the foot is pressed correctly into the floor.[59] The final aspect of the exercise, which involves lifting one leg, builds the primary thigh abductors.[60] Development of the muscles of the front of the leg, particularly the tibialis anterior, is essential for correctly executing the basic pivot and body rotation from the Box Stance. This pivot, which occurs throughout the Form, depends upon lifting (dorsiflexing) the foot and using the heel as the pivot point, while the knees may be in a deep state of flexion equivalent to the Chinese Horse Stance. This is necessary to execute a smooth and continuous transfer of weight to the opposite leg and to correctly transfer energy and power to the arms and hands. Properly done, this pivot exemplifies the principle "Energy is rooted in the feet, stems in the legs, is commanded by the waist, and functions through the fingers."

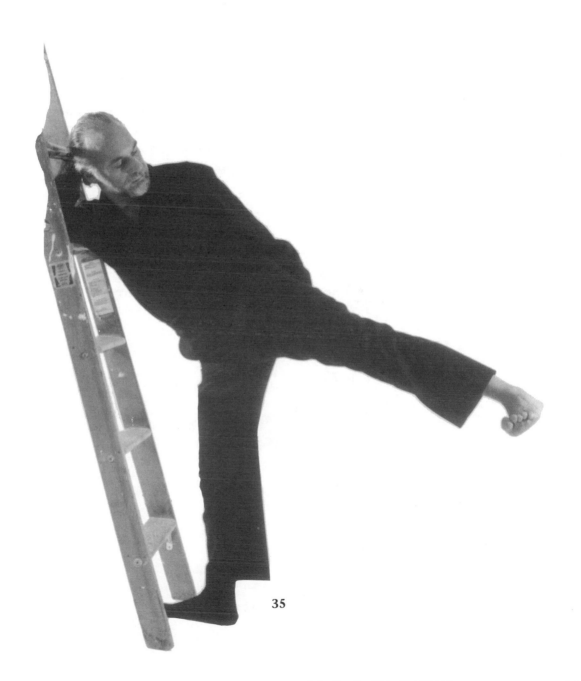

35

We have adapted two basic ballet exercises to both help stretch the groin and to facilitate balance. The first is the basic technique called First Position. I will describe it with the details of stretch that we have added to the position. The second is a variation of what is called in ballet the Fourth Position.

13. First Position.

Stand near a wall, or other object, to touch for balance if necessary. Bring the legs together and turn the feet out to the side. The toes should be pointing as close to 180 degrees apart as possible (Photo 36). The knees are

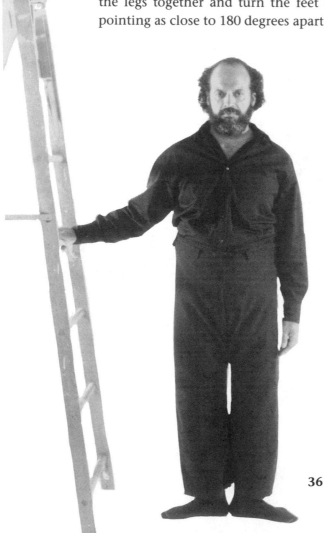

36

straight but not hyperextended. The thighs and knees should be in contact. Now you must attend carefully to the area of the *tan tien.* Using the gluteal muscles (the buttocks), pull the groin open. The anus must be relaxed, as in all T'ai Chi practice, but in this case the buttocks must tense to pull the groin. This is, for anyone with reasonable background, a most subtle exercise. It may take time to develop the awareness necessary to actually feel connections of the muscles, and even to feel the groin opening. If this is the case, the exercise is doubly important; as the area of the body in question is the center, the *tan tien,* the place where attention is to be focused always, it behooves the practitioner to do everything possible to feel it.

Open the knees out to the side as much as possible and slowly lower the body, while maintaining the T'ai Chi posture, and continue to stretch the groin and inner thighs. When the heels begin to raise, lift them and stretch so that only the area of the foot directly behind the toes is supporting the weight. The lower leg and foot are perfectly straight, with only the joints at the toes bent (Photo 37). This is a plié, except for the extreme lifting of the foot. Repeat a few times.

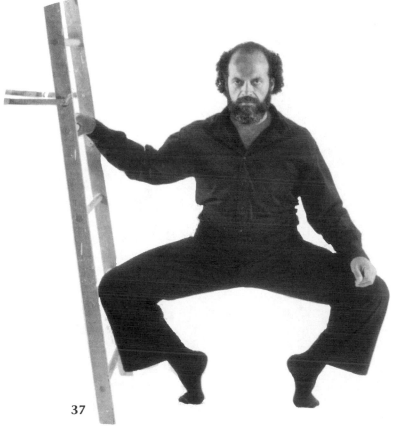

37

14. Modified Fourth Position.

Place the feet in the same starting position. Now move the right foot in front of the left so that the right heel is touching the left toe and the right toe is touching the left heel. Move the right foot forward about 8 inches and maintain the alignment (Photo 38). Slowly lower into a plié, attending to the following details. Make sure the knees are turned out as far apart as possible, and correct the feet to angle no more than the knees. Lift the heels as high as possible, once they are forced to raise off the floor. Keep the weight *forward* over the front heel and try to maintain the T'ai Chi posture (Photo 39). Repeat a few times.

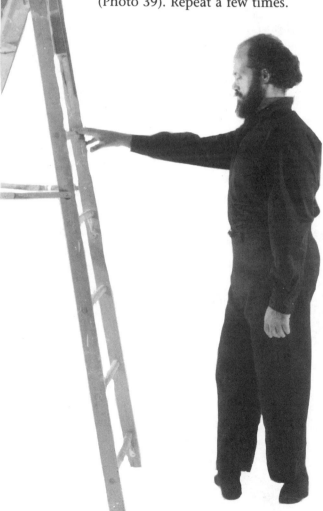

38

In the starting position of the first exercise, hip extension is produced by tucking the pelvis under and forward, forcing the groin open. Tucking the pelvis under is produced by tightening the gluteal muscles, while pulling the pubic bone up towards the navel and tilting the pelvis back. As the gluteal muscles are tightened, the adductor muscles of the groin and pelvic area are opened and stretched.[61]

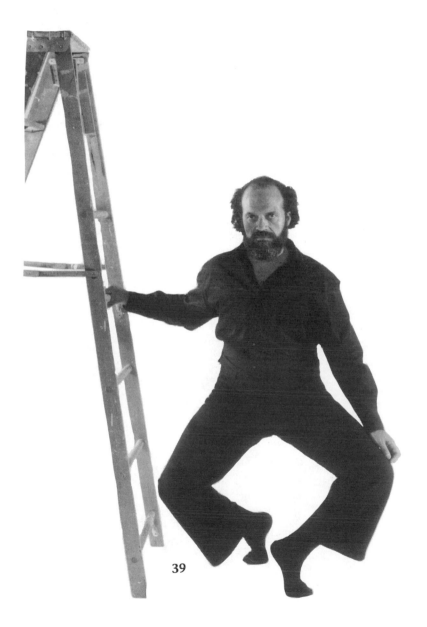

39

There is a tendency to release the tuck of the pelvis as the knees are flexed. The knees will also tend to rotate medially, if a concentrated effort is not made to hold the correct position. The quadricep muscles and the calf muscles,[62] which are supporting the body weight, are also stretched.

The fourth ballet position concentrates and increases the stretch and muscle development in these same muscle groups. It will improve the balance and the groin stretch needed to accomplish the more difficult stretch and balance movements in the Form, such as Carry Tiger Back to Mountain and Fairlady Works at Shuttles.

9
Postural Technique

THE T'AI CHI CHUAN FORM constitutes one of the most effective methods of producing alignment of the psychic centers and maintaining that alignment in motion. This is accomplished by a constant and vigilant effort to maintain and perfect a series of postures and transitions, while moving with strict adherence to principles. Of course, it is understood that strict adherence to principles is the constant observation of the process and the rapid and constant correction of all deviations. Intent is very important when working with energy and body retraining. This should not be misunderstood as justifying good intentions which are never realized. I mean that during the execution of the Form and in Push Hands, and hopefully in everyday life, the T'ai Chi Chuan practitioner is mindful of the proper execution of all movements and activities and corrects any observed errors instantly and constantly, without emotional reaction. Although it is possible to gain some degree of skill in T'ai Chi Chuan without serious study of posture and energy movement and control, the skills thus obtained are primarily a function of sensitivity and body dynamics and are much more akin to many styles of Kung Fu which remain external and do not seek to develop the control of Qi.

Postural Correction

We begin with the most fundamental and yet most virtually ignored aspect of postural correction: spinal realignment. A scientific rationale can be given for this, based upon the observation of animal spines, which are considerably straighter than that of man. With his upright stance, man has developed the so-called natural curvature of the spine as a result of gravity acting on his improper posture. With this postural misalignment, tremendous strength is sacrificed. The principles of T'ai Chi Chuan are based on the experimentally verifiable premise that the realignment of the spine, with combined modifications of certain states, will allow a free flow of Qi in the energy channels in the spine. This is the equivalent of Hatha Yoga spinal exercises used to produce a proper meditation posture, which culminates in the very difficult Bound Lotus.[63]

We will use the words referred to below as follows: *Belly* always refers to the area below the navel; *Stomach* always refers to the area above the navel. *Hollow* means to empty or hollow the area of muscle tension; *Fill* means to fill the area with the Qi from the opposing Hollow.

Many, many people pull in their stomachs for aesthetic purposes, while their back remains arched. This results in exactly the opposite energy effect desired in T'ai Chi Chuan, in which we must *fill* the lower back while *hollowing* the stomach (Fig. 6).

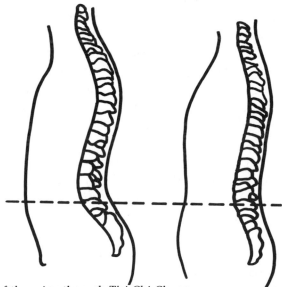

FIG. 6. Proper realignment of the spine through T'ai Chi Chuan

Spinal straightening is accomplished gradually through the attempt, at least during the execution of the Form, to hold the following posture. (Of course, the more time spent in properly holding the posture, the more natural and habitual it will become and the more rapidly will progress be made.)

TAO AND T'AI CHI KUNG

1. Plant the feet squarely, approximately shoulder-width apart, with the midline of the feet parallel and the weight evenly distributed over the bottom of each foot. Be careful not to take too wide of a stance. I have noticed that most people judge the width of their shoulders from the outside of the upper arms. In fact the width of the shoulder should be considered as slightly more than the width of the chest at the armpits.

2. Loosen the joints—let no joint be locked or stiffened; thus the ankles, knees, and the juncture of the legs and trunk at the groin *must* be bent. There is a strong tendency to lean back and thrust the hips forward, thereby locking the joint at the juncture of the legs and trunk. This makes it impossible to properly root or control Qi. Always, even when bending backward and dropping, if you are strongly pushed down in Push Hands, you must not let the leg/torso joint straighten and lock. This should be carefully considered if you wish great skill in combative activities.

3. Fill the lower belly and relax the perineum and buttocks. (This concept will be further developed and explained in relation to the *tan tien*.)

4. Hollow the upper abdomen from the sternum to the navel. As you do so, the lower back should fill up and the lumbar curve should become straight. To accomplish this, try placing your thumb against the upper tip of the sternum and stretch the hand so that the little finger is in contact with the navel. Try to shorten the distance between your fingers without sliding them; that is, move or drop your sternum down toward your belly. This will help with dropping the ribcage and therefore should be done in conjunction with the next step.

5. Drop the rib cage. This further facilitates straightening of the back; it also reduces the tension and helps sink the body weight back onto the legs and into the ground. Usually the lower portion of the rib cage tends to have an outward flare, and if you place your hand along the rib cage from chest to stomach, you will probably notice this outward flare. As you do the exercise described in Step 4, you should notice the rib cage change so that it curves inward. At this point, one of the more difficult aspects of breaking years and years of wrong habits becomes apparent: As you hollow the stomach and drop the

ribs, your upper body and head will tend to curve forward, increasing the difficulty of the next part of the posture. Yet all aspects of the posture must be accomplished together if real progress is to be made. This is also the point where one of the more radical changes in appearance of the body takes place, especially for the American male with his desire for a V-shaped, or "chesty" look. This is a process of simply relaxing muscles that are locked into unnatural tension. The position of the rib cage must change as shown in the photo on the next page.

6. Open the shoulders. Man tends to produce what we like to call "the turtle effect" as a result of the psychological withdrawal described in the section "Man's Tension as Psychic Armor." The shoulders are usually pulled up and forward, producing a hunched back (additional spinal curvature), a forward-tilted neck, improper weight distribution, etc. To correct this, the shoulders should first be lifted up without strain, while keeping the arms relaxed, then *rotated* back (so that the elbows point to the rear), pulled down using the muscles of the back as described in The Cross Exercise (see page 90), and relaxed (eventually) into that position. In time, this will become the natural position of your shoulders, and the shoulder blades should return to their normal flat position, instead of protruding.

   Remember that the progression above must be accomplished without sacrificing the lower and mid-body postural corrections. You will find that Steps 1 to 5 usually can be accomplished and maintained together; when you do this step, you will probably find that you have lost most of the first five steps. This is the result of the incorrect postures that we have all been taught to hold since we walked into our first public school physical education class.[64] You will need to repeat Step 1 to 5 and then 6 (and 7) and struggle to control the positions obtained by constant repetition, until the "feel" of the combination is developed. Remember that this is not simple exercise. You are retraining a lifetime of incorrect posture and tension. It will take time. If you persist, the reward will be much greater than you expect.

7. Straighten the neck. This aspect of postural change is in many ways the most difficult technique of T'ai Chi Chuan. It is,

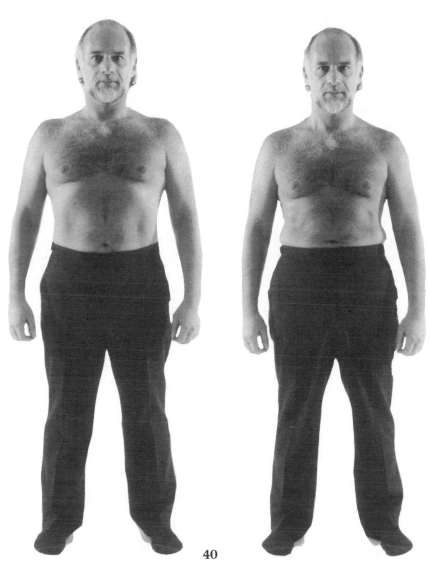

40

Normal lifted ribcage posture   Proper T'ai Chi Chuan posture

however, absolutely necessary if one is involved in the esoteric aspect of energy development. If this is not accomplished, martial art skills as well as general health can still be developed to a reasonable degree. However, to accomplish the free flow of energy or "The Self-Turning Wheel of the Law," it is imperative that the neck be straightened for the final alignment of the psychic centers. It is also necessary to straighten the neck to obtain both the maximum physical health and martial art skills.

Activating the Qi in T'ai Chi Chuan   109

When the Qi flows freely, the general health begins to improve. With concentration of the energy, various other abilities can become manifest, such as the ability to increase ancestral Qi in the chest for power and health. Eventually the "Qi of Prior Heaven," which is fixed at birth and lost throughout life, can be replenished, increasing longevity considerably.[65]

As a result of the many unhealthy deviations in correct human posture, coupled with an attitude of curiosity—often physically manifest as a jutting head—man's neck is unnaturally curved and protruded forward; the head is tilted back, resulting in a very blocked energy system.

In conjunction with the shoulder movement described in Step 6, the following should be accomplished. Drop the head back and then "pull it up" from behind, as the chin is lowered toward the interclavicular notch (the hollow spot in the middle of the clavicle). Lowering the chin is very important and should produce an intense sensation of pulling at the back of the neck. A tendon should stand out on the back of the neck to the thickness of perhaps a ¼ to a ½ inch and should gradually become very tight and hard. Slowly, after a period of time, this tension will decrease and the tendon will soften. This tension results from poor neck posture, which tends to produce foreshortening of the muscles at the back of the neck (Fig. 7).[66]

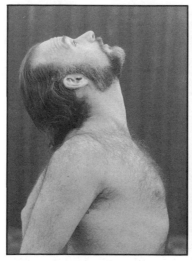 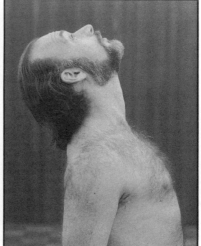

In addition, there is usually a sensation of constriction (even choking) in the throat, perhaps a sore throat and swollen glands in the front of the neck. If you practice every day for two to four weeks, that will pass and the neck posture will be correct (Fig. 8). *Warning:* Do not continue to hold the head and neck in the new posture should you begin to have a headache at the base of the skull. As soon as you feel more than stretching discomfort, *stop* and start again later that day, or the next day.

8. Align the teeth and jaws by properly aligning the incisors and minimizing the overlap of the top teeth. Touch the tip of the tongue to the palate just behind the incisors. The chin has been lowered slightly by the neck straightening, so you must lift the eyes to look straight ahead. This should produce an awareness of the bony ridge above the eyes. This posture allows the proper circulation of Qi in both the external and internal pathways, along the *du* and *ren* channels described earlier. The superficial or external circulation simply makes a circuit along the midline of the body, flowing down the torso in the front (which is not the normal direction of the *ren* channel), through *tan tien,* up the spine, over the head and face, where it can be felt to tingle in the teeth as it passes down. The more important deep circulation follows a similar pathway but is experienced quite differently; it travels more deeply in the head and face. As it

FIG. 7. Unlocking the energy in the neck

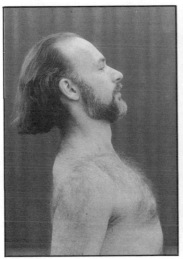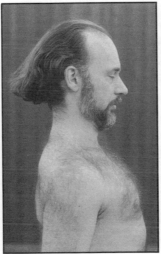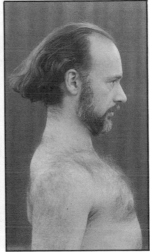

passes through the Third Eye center deep between the eyebrows, it divides into two channels along the orbital ridge of the eyes, then down through the cheeks where it reunites at the palate and flows through the tongue as it passes down.

At this point, if all the postural efforts are made and the body properly held, there is proper alignment and the stage is set for the energy flow. Now we must turn to the single most important aspect of T'ai Chi Chuan, which is the development or opening of the *tan tien*.

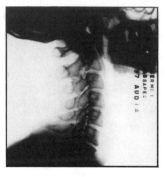 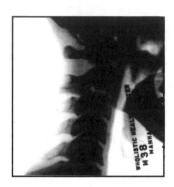

FIG. 8. Normal cervical vertebrae   T'ai Chi neck posture

Tan Tien: The Field of Healing

Three tenths of the distance from the navel to the pubic bone on the midline of the body lies a point known in Acupuncture as the Main Center of Energy. It is often called by practitioners of Aikido the One Point. This point is, in fact, the place through which the energy can be stimulated for rebalancing certain systemic energetic imbalances. It is the access point to the *tan tien* and can be used in meditation as a primary point of focus. However, this is not really the *tan tien,* although many think, and rightly so, that through long and conscientious meditation on that point, that psychic center can be opened.

The opening of the *tan tien* is, however, a far more physically complex—although far less time consuming—process in the practice of T'ai Chi Chuan. In theory, one who practices properly twice daily (20 minutes each time) for three years will open the *tan tien.* Many years of serious meditation will be required to accomplish the same task by sitting and meditating on the point of access to the *tan tien,* or the One Point.

The opening of the *tan tien* is in fact the primary goal of T'ai Chi Chuan. When it opens, progress in self-development and the development of Teh can proceed rapidly. Physical health improves dramatically and the use of awkward muscle strength becomes quite archaic in light of the new powers of relatively free-flowing Qi. *Tan tien* literally means "field of medicine" (actually a *tan* is a medicinal pill), implying an area that is a source of medicine or healing. Physical, emotional, mental, and most important, spiritual health can be gained from the proper opening of *tan tien* and subsequent activation of the conservation and transformation functions that have their origin there. This is the place of the first of the three cauldrons in which the spiritual child is nurtured. Even before that occurs, it is the place from which the initial energy activation occurs in the superficial circulation that eventually allows the head centers to be prepared for the deeper circulation. On a more superficial level, the Chinese *tan tien* is exactly the same as the Japanese *hara*—the "belly," the physically-rooted center from which all things can grow unperturbed. As my T'ai Chi Master Ahn loved to point out, the great religious art of India, Japan, China, and Tibet, at the height of their artistic and spiritual civilizations, always showed the gods in the formal T'ai Chi posture with perfectly straight back and neck and flat stomach, with the belly protruding below the navel. This is a reversal of the ego-inflating posture of the West, where the belly and stomach are pulled in and up, and the groin and buttocks tensed.

The general tension of the lower digestive tract has led to a nation of people who live on laxatives and pain-killers. Chronic constipation and faulty digestion through tension can be causally related to a tremendous number of diseases which torture people, including the common cold which, many have heard their doctor say, disappears or lessens with a healthy bowel movement. Thus, the effort to open the *tan tien* is probably one of the most positive efforts toward health that Americans can make. To master *tan tien* is to reverse the unnatural aging process of people in the modern world. Yet the technique seems to be a touchy subject and is generally avoided, even in books on *hara* of Japan. What follows is, to my relatively extensive knowledge of the literature (in English) of T'ai Chi Chuan and the *Hara*-centered Japanese art of Aikido, the first detailed description of the physical technique of opening the *tan tien.*

"Let go" is the key. Let go to the force of gravity, let go of your chest, let go of your stomach, stop pulling it in and making it tight while pulling your chest up. A student once commented on her first experience of seeing the formal posture compared to the "normal" posture: "It sure isn't sexy!" Although she was stating a personal aesthetic opinion, what she didn't know is that one's sexual energy is considerably increased through *tan tien* mastery.

The whole abdominal area is covered with a muscular sheath called the rectus abdominus, which is divided into several segments by horizontal bands of ligament—two above, one at, and one below the navel. One ligament called the linea alba runs vertically down the center. These ligaments combined produce the "wash-board" stomach of body builders. A smaller muscle, the pyramidalis, covers the rectus abdominus at the pubic bone and attaches to the linea alba, which it tightens. We must learn to relax and protrude the lower portion of the rectus abdominus as well as the pyramidalis, while relaxing and hollowing the upper portion of the rectus abdominus. When the belly is relaxed, the chest and spine aligned, and the internal organs returned to their rightful lower place, this allows for the hollowing of the stomach and the filling of the belly without muscle tension.

Although the "full belly" is the *tan tien,* we must develop a three-dimensional sense about this body, and not cling to the surface protrusion. So, to relax the belly means not only to let go of the rectus abdominus, but the pyramidalis and all muscles of the groin, the buttocks, and the perineum. Thus, we summarize the *tan tien* as follows (this description constitutes the first posture of T'ai Chi Chuan, called Wu Chi or the Void, from which it all begins):

1. Set the feet parallel and shoulder-width apart. Distribute the weight evenly on the bottom surface of the feet.
2. Bend all the joints.
3. Fill the belly; hollow the stomach; straighten the lower back.
4. Relax the buttocks, the anus, and the genitals.
5. Pull the shoulders back and down and sink the rib cage.
6. Straighten the neck.
7. Align the teeth and touch the palate with the tongue.
8. "Look up" from under your eyebrows.
9. Relax, let go, give up control—be one with the heaven above and the earth below. You are suspended from the crown of your head—with your bones aligned. Gravity suppports you. You are an energy channel. Let the energy flow and work for you. Observe.

Points 3 and 4 cannot be over-emphasized. These are very difficult but extremely essential aspects of T'ai Chi Chuan and *tan tien* development. People tend, for reasons of appearance, to tighten and pull in the whole abdomen and, because of various emotional and psychological tensions, to "clench" all the sphincters (circular muscles that close orifices) in the area of the perineum. The first results of the practice, if the relaxation is accomplished, is a feeling of vulnerability, of "openness," which soon turns into a feeling of what I will describe as "happy freedom" for want of a better expression. In the early stages of practice, this relaxation should be the focus of attention.

The sense of vulnerability is most easily overcome by the practice of the Form. With consistent practice of the posture, by the time one begins Push Hands, one should have already begun to experience the opening of the *tan tien* area.

The *tan tien* is the center. All movement in T'ai Chi Chuan should come from the center. Body movement is initiated with the belly and extends into the legs and torso. The arm movements must be coordinated so that there is as little independent limb movement as possible. The arms are an extension of the torso and thus should only continue its movement. The T'ai Chi movements are such that the body, moving quickly, can in fact throw the arms into the approximate positions they take during the Form. It is very difficult to explain many T'ai Chi Chuan principles, and the hint given above will, in time, allow you to discover the truth pragmatically.

The technique whereby the *tan tien* is opened and the weight let down is collectively referred to as *sinking*. Throughout the practice of T'ai Chi Chuan, the practitioner is constantly trying to relax into each posture, to let go of the upward pull of his musculature, to sink. Sinking produces rooting, an attachment to the earth, a unifying of the energy of the practitioner and the surface. Rooting makes one immovable—rooting makes one psychologically freer.

Conclusion

The Wu Chi is Eternal—Heaven and Earth pass away but the Supreme *is*. The T'ai Chi, the Ultimate Tao, is patient, for it is infinite. The practitioner must be patient to be in accord with the Tao. The T'ai Chi, the Ultimate Tao, is persistent for it is infinite. The practitioner must be persistent, to be in accord with the Tao. The T'ai Chi, the Ultimate Tao, does not hurry, for it is infinite. The practitioner must not hurry, to be in accord with the Tao — then he will have Teh. Practice with a sense of slowness. Wait until you are balanced. Wait until the energy moves you. Wait.

.

Appendix

Some Comments on Written Language and Chinese

I would like to explain two problems which cause certain misunderstandings to arise, especially for those whose major interests lie in martial arts and not in Chinese studies in general. One problem lies in the lack of true appreciation for the dynamic nature of both written and spoken language in general. The other problem lies with those subtle and usually unexpressed distinctions that make apparently identical ideas in different cultures have very different meanings and carry very different emotional attachments.

The history of written language is the fascinating study of man's struggle to expand and evolve his mind far beyond the limits of his animal nature. It is common knowledge that many animals use various means of communication beyond audible cries and calls. We all know odors are used extensively in the animal kingdom to mark territories and inform intruders of their errors, much as men post No Trespassing signs. Wild horses mark their domains with "stud piles" produced at will upon the approach of an intruder. Elaborate, individualized claw marks on trees define the domain of Far Eastern hunting tigers, reminiscent of the monograms used by humans to mark their property. City street gangs use icons drawn on the ground, or "tags" (monogram-like gang names) scrawled on walls to mark their territories. Many cities, probably due to the multilingual character that they have developed, increasingly use descriptive icons to replace written instructions for traffic signs. Many thousands of years ago, as a result of the evolving complexity of even so-called primitive societies, men began to develop more sophisticated use of markings or written symbols primarily for inventory and accountkeeping purposes. As man, forced by circumstances, began to seek fuller and more complex communications with his fellows, simple numerical accounting gave way to pictures used as reminders of a message, song, or story that had already been set to memory. Reminding sticks, scribed with simple icons, are still in use today among tribes in Africa and South America. With time and need, the early pictograms[67] appear to have evolved into complex written communication forms.[68] Although the Chinese written language initially evolved as we have outlined, it developed into a much more sophisticated vehicle of communication.

The icons that make up the written Chinese language are used in three different ways. Many are simple pictograms depicting the objects of common interest. The basic icons are then combined; additional strokes (of the writing brush) may be added, to form more complex icons, and thereby imply more complex meanings. Since Chinese is essentially a monosyllabic language, the addition of a phonogram symbol to the pictogram completes the word, providing both a picture and a sound to represent it. Because the complex results of combining icons lead beyond representations of objects and simple action verbs, the Chinese language is capable of expressing sophisticated and profound *ideas.* Therefore we call its individual characters *ideograms* in recognition of the profound distinction between the functions of the icons used in inventory and accounts and memory jogging, and those used for philosophy in the Chinese language. When reading ancient Chinese writings, we must remember that we are reading a grouping of pictures that represented an abstract idea to a thinker in an entirely different time, place, culture, value system, and belief system. It is very easy to impose our own ideas and the values and beliefs of our culture on old documents that are difficult to understand. If you look at detailed translations of ancient texts, you will quickly agree that there is little that is really understood, and much that is clearly "guessed" or imposed on the ancient authors.

In Chapter 1, we analyzed one of the ancient Chinese characters, *Teh,* and I hope this has been accomplished without imposing modern-day views. At the same time, as the meaning of the ancients may not be valuable in the modern world if translated directly, it is necessary to find the essence of the idea, and clothe it in modern garb. To use a profound and significant example from the *Tao Teh Ching,* we can look at the admonition by Lao Tze to "accept disgrace willingly." Most modern Western people would smile and shrug off any significance in such behavior. In traditional Chinese culture, reputation was generally more significant than life itself. Although to this day suicide is a valid way of saving face in the minds of thousands of young university failures in Japan each year, saving face is not really a factor in the minds of modern Western people. However, if we can find a concept that is able to produce the exact same response in a modern young Westerner as "accept disgrace willingly" did in Lao Tze's ancient Chinese listeners, we will have found a valid translation. Because the modern seeker of the same path in the West has grown up in a culture in which independence, self-assertion, and civil disobedience have become more important than life itself, we can simply alter the literal meaning to express the intended meaning, "accept authority willingly." In making this studied modification, we have imposed a task of equal magnitude on the modern independent youth.[69]

One other aspect of the language, or perhaps more an aspect of the Chinese culture, is the rather broad variety of names applied to a single person. Given and surnames are not often used. The name that is used by a person, or used in reference to that person, may differ under differing circumstances. Finally, there is often a title or a descriptive appellation which, in common usage, usurps the real name of the individual. Further English corruption complicates the situation. *Confucius* is a good example of this total corruption. For many years I thought Confucius was someone's actual name. It is, in fact, a linguistic corruption of the descriptive appellation *Kung Fu Tze,* The Philosopher of the Result of Right Action. It is also important to remember that in many cases the ancients could be mythical figures painted as allegorical extremes for the purpose of influencing young minds, i.e., moral education. In Chapter 1, we used both aspects in assessing the implications of the words of Lao Tze.

Endnotes

Chapter 1: Introduction to the Fundamentals of Taoist Thought

1. Many have come to teach the Way of Enlightenment and few, if any, have felt that they were able to accomplish any significant result. Jesus said, "What can we say of this generation. . .we piped and they would not dance, we played but they would not sing. . . .And John came neither eating nor drinking and they said he had a demon, and the Son of Man came both eating and drinking and they called him a glutton and a winebibber." (Matthew 11:16-17) G.I. Gurdjieff, in his magnificent work *All and Everything,* describes a succession of cosmic messengers over eons of time who are all disappointed in their efforts to bring enlightenment to mankind on any significant scale. Gurdjieff reminds us that the work of returning to the Absolute source is going against the general stream of "descent from the Absolute" and therefore is only possible for very small numbers of people. Lao Tze departed feeling the same frustration.

2. Since there was a 500 year period between the times of these philosophers, this is obviously not an accurate historical event. It is an anecdote created to show how far Lao Tze's thinking was from the traditional Chinese view of the way to think about the world and man's relationship to it.

3. The words esoteric and exoteric here are used as in spiritual and philosophical writings. Esoteric philosophies are not the same as occult philosophies or practices. Occult refers to those practices that grow out of science and are aimed toward control of metaphysical forces. Esoteric refers to those ideas that grow out of philosophy and are aimed toward wisdom and transcendence. They are "hidden" and traditionally revealed only to those deemed ready. Exoteric refers to the ideas freely given which lead to the deeper thoughts. The teachings of the Christian, Hebrew, and Islamic churches are exoteric. The teachings of their respective secretive and mystical branches—the Gnostics, the "Doctors of the Law," and the Sufis—are esoteric.

4. From the *Tantra Shastra,* the basic texts of the highly maligned Tantra Yoga.

5. In Gyana Yoga, the Yoga of Knowledge, attainment is realized through knowing and embracing the true nature of Reality. Its teachings are closely connected to the Taoist phrase "Ever desireless, one can see the mystery."

6. This is a basic idea unrelated to Einstein's work on relativity. The point of Einstein's theory was not to demonstrate that which was already known but to show that the

speed (usually relative motion) of light was *not relative* in our experiential universe and that it was in fact the only referential constant in this universe.

7. For the scientific viewpoint see, *The Dancing Wu Li Masters.* The esoteric philosophical position of P.D. Ouspensky is expressed in his original works *A New Model of the Universe* and *Tertium Organum,* but it is brought to fruition by his work with G.I. Gurdjieff, which is documented in Ouspensky's greatest work, *In Search of the Miraculous.*

8. Throughout this book, certain sentences will appear in italics. These are sentences that can form the basis of meaningful meditations and can be valuable if pondered. By meditation I mean the cognitive process of "unpacking" the complex idea expressed in the sentence. This is a process used in the philosophical discipline of linguistic analysis, the methodology of Ludwig Wittgenstein. One of the most intelligent and highly evolved examples of such a meditation is the book *The Concept of Mind* by Gilbert Ryle. A more realistic set of examples can be found in *The Meditations of Marcus Aurelius.*

9. The philosophies of India agree that Earth is the lowest level; yogic texts show the Primal Shakti, in her form as the Serpent Goddess, descending through increasingly dense manifestion worlds until she rests in the *Bhu loka* or Earth plane. The yogi tries to activate the Goddess in his lowest chakra and bring her to ascend with him, through progressively less phenomenal worlds, back to the source. In G. Gurdjieff's method of enlightenment, called the Fourth Way, the Moon is seen as a denser, more law-bound reality; it draws energy from the life of the Earth, and man, under the Moon's influence, deteriorates.

10. George Harrison sings it, *Om purnamadah purnamidam. Purnat purnamudacyate. Purnasya purnamadaya. Purnamevavashishyate.* (Invocation from the Iso-upanishad; see *The Upanishads,* by Swami Nikhilananda, Vol. 1, Harper and Brothers Publishers, 1949.)

11. John 1:5

12. Remember that the things of Heaven are Yin and Yang to each other, and the things of Earth are Yin and Yang to each other; but all things of Heaven are Yang and all things of Earth are Yin in the relation *between* Heaven and Earth.

13. This has never been the true scientific view. Although many scientists, in reaction to the phantasamagoria of the Dark Ages, were scrupulously non-religious and non-mystical in their writings, it is in the writings of Arthur Eddington, James Jeans, Albert Einstein, et al. that the mystic shows through in the great scientist. In modern physics, the ideas of esoteric philosophy have found new champions. I recommend reading *The Dancing Wu Li Masters,* which effectively introduces the ideas of waves of probability and the need for a conscious observer, and other "unscientific" truths of modern science.

14. Most of the modern writers on evolution hold that either natural selection or survival of the fittest is the only cause of evolutionary change. Since philosophers, mystics, and artists would, in a natural environment, be the least likely to produce great numbers of offspring and the least likely to survive any inter- or intra-tribal conflicts, the level of such activities among so-called primitive and ancient peoples is astounding.

15. From the *Brihadaranyaka Upanishad.*

16. The terms idea and ideal, although not really the same, seem to be used almost interchangeably by philosophers when speaking of Plato's ideas. His World of Ideas, it could be said, are the ideas of ideal reality.

17. The Ideal Man of Plato can be equated with the Adam Kadman, or Universal Man of mystical Judaism. The Hebrews, however, saw the Universal Man as the sum of

the souls of mankind, both before and after the ages pass, and they did not see individual men as expressions attempting to emulate the ideal.

18. Peter Tompkins and Christoper Bird, *The Secret Life of Plants*, New York: Avon Books, 1973; p. 31.

19. Ibid, p. 35.

20. Non-dualist Truth, the *Bharata Dharma* (philosophy of India), includes a hierarchy of philosophical positions starting with pure materialism and evolving through dualistic philosophy (yogic dualism) into monism and ultimately the non-dualist Truth. Brahman, according to Advaite Vedanta, is the source of all that is, but all that is exists only as illusion. There is no world, but only Brahman, who is eternally possessed of the quality of *maya*, artistic expression, which is also called *lila*, the divine dance.

Chapter 2: Practical Examples of Li and Qi

21. In Taoist works, man is often considered a three-centered being. In Fourth Way work, we call him a seven-centered being. According to yogic vision, he has 144 psychic centers, each of which has a particular function. The Buddhists work with twelve. In yoga, we usually work with seven. There are three that are fundamental: the Head center, the Heart or chest center, and the Belly or body center. When we speak of the Head center at this stage, we are speaking of the reflection of the Mind into the world, or Personality, which resides "at the surface," as it were, of the body (see Chart 3).

Chapter 3: Application of the Principle of Li to T'ai Chi Chuan

22. The fascinating study of body types (Sheldon, W. *The Varieties of Human Physique and the Varieties of Temperment*), and the odd mixes they produce, can be extremely useful in understanding fundamental behaviors and motivation in human activity.

23. This is explained at the beginning of Patanjali's Yoga Aphorisms. (See James H. Woods, *The Yoga System of Patanjali.*)

Chapter 4: Acquiring Control of Qi

24. It is strange that Western man tends to reject those invisible forces that he himself can control, while electricity, magnetism, gravity, gamma rays from space, and waves of energy measured in the brain and used in biofeedback—all the stuff that our science is made of—is invisible and accepted. Yet the Qi of Acupuncture and T'ai Chi is summarily rejected by the very ones who seek to build gigantic and expensive cyclotrons to accelerate the invisible particles seen only as trails in smoke. Is there not clearly an irrational prejudice here?

25. Tina Sohn is a Diagnostic Sensitive, one who literally feels the total physical and psychological condition of another by contact. A more literal term would be "empath"; she refuses, however, to allow the ability to manifest outside of her health care practice. Her book, *Amma: The Ancient Art of Oriental Healing* (Healing Arts Press) gives a background of her training in childhood and accounts for the unnerving abilities that she had already acquired when we met in Korea. I was more than double her weight and yet she would say, "Oh, I'm so heavy, I can't hold myself up, help me!" I could not, no matter what I attempted in response, get her feet to

leave the ground. It took me more than ten years of intense effort before I could actually overcome her root.

26. The Du and Ren Mo, the conception and governing vessels respectively, are important channels that traverse the midline of the body along the front and back respectively. In addition to being of great import in the treatment of disease, they form, when properly cultivated, a continuous flow of Qi, down the front, up the back, and over the head. This basic flow of Qi is necessary for all advanced forms of spiritual development. In the practice of Indian Yoga, the development of Qi flow is often forced with dangerous results; the great master Ramakrishna even blamed his early excesses in *pranayama* (energy control exercises) for his later throat cancer. In Chinese Yoga this flow is accomplished passively through postural correction and slow deliberate movement to guide the Qi, which is T'ai Chi Chuan; the forced breathing and internal muscular locks of Indian Yoga are abjured. Once this flow has evolved to a point where it is self-sustaining, it is called The Self-Turning Wheel of the Law. Then the practice of specific Qi Kung exercises leads to further advanced energy manipulation.

Chapter 5: The Mind and the Balance of the Body

27. This is the point called Kidney 1 in Acupuncture. The Kidney channel contains the driving Qi of all the channels. It also connects to the Extraordinary channels, which have a deeper energetic significance; it is believed that they carry the prenatal Qi, which activates all that occurs. This prenatal Qi cannot be replenished by ordinary means, although it can be dissipated rapidly by excess and incontinence. As it ebbs, life ebbs. Its end is the end of life. Nei Kung exercises, including T'ai Chi Chuan, can replenish it.

28. It seems to be the same principle that underlies any developmental process—the seeing of continuity and unity in whatever you're dealing with.

29. Something that you could find quite useful to do when you read, if you do not already do so, is to stop and picture the image that the author presents and to contemplate the implications of the image. Most people would read this and not stop; they would wonder what the author is talking about or they would be pleased by the pretty image and not bother to go on to the implications of the idea, to try to see and feel what that means in the body.

30. Chinese medical philosophy describes seven souls in man which are correlated to specific organ complexes. *Shen,* the soul residing in the Heart, represents our general concept of emotional drives, desires, and needs (not including physical needs).

31. The things of Heaven are Yin and Yang, yet all are Yang relative to Earth. In the same way, the lower torso is generally substantial and the upper insubstantial. While the supporting leg is substantial and the other leg is insubstantial, the attacking arm, hand, and side are substantial while the yielding arm, hand, and side are insubstantial.

Chapter 6: Some Important Principles of T'ai Chi Chuan

32. For an explanation of the nature and cause of gastric ptosis and other conditions, see Barral and Mercier, *Visceral Manipulation,* pp. 121-123.

33. The technique called Poison Hand is one of the most esoteric and difficult of the martial arts. It is the art of striking specific energy loci with light force to obtain dramatic results. The practitioner may cause mild pain, severe neurological distur-

bance, severe pathology, or even delayed death.

34. I discuss the process of development of the emotional and intellectual centers in my books *On Willingness To Be Wrong* and *On Transcendental Aim*. For the general process as described in Ashtanga Yoga, with emphasis on emotional development through *yama* and *niyama*, see *The Reality of Living Yoga*.

Chapter 7: Benefits of Practicing the Form

35. This refers to what is called "listening energy," the ability to know what your opponent is doing in his most subtle movements; to know his imbalances, his tension, his intentions—in short, to hear his Qi. We can also speak of "sticking energy," "leading energy," and other forms of special awareness acquired through the hands. These are advanced Push Hands techniques which we will cover in a future text.

36. A clear example of this lies in Chinese medical philosophy, which attempts to force every phenomena into the limits of the Five Elements. Thus we have the five viscera, five bowels, five tissues, five seasons, five emotions, etc., all related very specifically as the "correspondences," which is one of the main theoretical bases for Acupuncture. Clearly there are more than five of any of the above mentioned subjects, with the exception of seasons which generally number four. It is to the credit of the practitioners of Chinese medicine that, through "creative manipulation" of such concepts relative to observation, phenomenal results are obtained in the treatment of disease.

Chapter 8: Adjunct Exercises

37. This includes the pectineus, adductor longus and brevis, adductor magnus, and the gracilis muscles.

38. This area is primarily comprised of the tendons of the quadriceps femoris group: rectus femoris, vastus intermedius, vastus medialis, and vastus lateralis.

39. See "Exercise-Induced Muscle Damage, Repair, and Adaptation in Humans," by P. Clarkson and I. Tremblay in *Journal of Applied Physiology,* V 65, no.1, July 1988.

40. Dr. Arnold Foster was responsible for starting me on my bonesetting studies and also kindled my interest in practicing Acupuncture. Prior to that, my interest was only in the area of energy control and the details of the energy conversion processes. I only applied Acupuncture as a healing art with students and family, specifically in relation to emotional difficulties that need to be overcome in spiritual work.

41. Especially the rectus abdominus, pyramidalis, and iliopsoas.

42. This includes the upper erector spinae, splenius capitis and cervicis, and trapezius.

43. This includes the erector spinae group (iliocostalis, longissimus, and spinalis) and the transversospinalis muscles, which lie beneath the erector spinae.

44. The biceps femoris, semitendinosus, and semimembranosus muscles.

45. The gastrocnemius, soleus, plantaris muscles.

46. The intervertebral ligaments, the posterior longitudinal ligament, the ligamentum flava, the nuchal ligament, and the interspinous ligaments are also stretched.

47. This includes the upper erector spinae, splenius capitis and cervicis, upper, middle and lower trapezius, middle and lower erector spinae, latissimus dorsi, and the quadratus lumborum.

48. This stretch starts at the throat with the platsyma and hyoid muscles. It lengthens the rectus abdominus, the linea alba (the ligament that runs through the rectus

abdominus), the pyramidalis, and the iliopsoas.

49. This motion produces a maximal stretch of the anterior longitudinal ligament (linea alba) and an opening of the anterior intervetebral disc spaces. As a result, the posterior joints of the spine (facets) and the spinous processes are gently compressed, helping to release toxic substances retained in the area.

50. This generally stretches the quadricep muscles of the thigh and maximally stretches the patella, anterior cruciate, and fibula collateral ligaments, the iliotibial tract, the muscles and tendons of the knee, including the popliteus, the lateral head of the gastrocnemius, and the biceps femoris.

51. This includes the tibialis anterior, extensor digitorum, extensor hallicus longus, and peroneus longus and brevis.

52. These include the rectus femoris, which is the only muscle of the quadricep group that crosses both the knee and hip. The ligaments of the patella and posterior cruciate are also significantly stretched.

53. Plantar flexion of the ankles brings the stretch to the anterolateral muscles of the legs and to the dorsal surface of the feet, affecting the tibialis anterior, the extensor digitorum, and the extensor hallicus longus.

54. This works the tibial colateral ligament, semimembranosis tendon (which inserts on the medial aspect of the knee), and the semitendinosis tendon (which inserts on the anterior aspect of the knee).

55. These protrude on many people because of weak rhomboids (muscles of the upper back that should hold the scapula flat.)

56. These attach the ischial tuberosity of the pelvis to the tibia and fibula (below the knee).

57. These attach the ilium and sacrum to the femur.

58. The gluteal muscles and tendons, the tensor fascia latae, and the iliotibial tract (which attach the femur to the pelvis) are stretched significantly.

59. By doing this, the peroneus tertius, longus, and brevis muscles and tendons, the posterior and anterior talofibular ligaments, and the calcaneofibular and talocalcaneal ligaments are all maximally stretched.

60. The gluteus medius and minimus muscles, as well as the iliopsoas, the tensor fascia latae, and the sartorius, which assist in this motion, are also strengthened.

61. An increase in the stretch at the medial knee should also be felt due to an increased pull on the sartorius muscle, as the iliac spines are rotated laterally. The sartorius muscle is attached to the iliac spines and inserts at the upper medial shaft of the tibia below the knee.

62. The gastrocnemius, soleus, and plantaris.

Chapter 9: Postural Technique

63. See page 84 for a description of the Lotus posture. Add the following modification after you have mastered the Lotus. Cross your arms behind your lower back and grasp the foot on each side with the opposite hand.

64. The horror of Physical Education was made clear to me in 1968, when I was teaching sixth grade in the New York Public School System. I had begun to teach Hatha Yoga techniques to my class, a form of exercise that they enjoyed and in which their young supple bodies were amazingly adept. After several of my colleagues observed this practice, I was visited by the District Supervisor of Physical Education and warned that if I did not cease and desist from these dangerous exercises that would permanently damage the children's joints, I would be brought up on charges and dismissed. I quit teaching that year.

65. The Taoist aim in working with Qi is quite clear. As the Qi is concentrated and circulated, it stimulates a number of psychic centers in turn, each having specific functions in producing the homonculus or spiritual child, which is nurtured and nourished in each of the three cauldrons, or three major centers previously discussed, until it is fully evolved. The yogi (Taoist in this case) then produces an adamantine body which is indestructible in this world; he continues with additional work until he is free of karmic residue and fully enlightened. He then dissolves into the Absolute (see Lu, *Taoist Yoga.*)

66. The condition of a straight neck or "military neck" is not desirable. Straight cervical vertebra, without the rest of the spinal column being straight, are a structural problem that require chiropractic manipulation. In T'ai Chi Chuan, the neck is straightened *along with* the thoracic and lumbar vertebrae.

Appendix

67. Pictograms (or pictographs) are icons—small pictures representing a particular object. A phonogram, on the other hand, is a phonetic element, representing a sound. In early language, phonograms evolved from the first sound of the pictogram, irrespective of the pictogram's meaning. For example, a picture of a horse as a pictograph would be read HORSE, but as a phonogram it would be the sound H.

68. Anyone interested in this fascinating subject will find references in the Selected Readings section. If you are not familiar with the work in this field, be prepared for a series of shocking revelations about the thought processes, prejudices, and fatuous self-righteousness of the many so-called great thinkers of the fifteenth through the eighteenth centuries. We have imposed so much, both more and less than was true, on the ancient writings that we have discovered. (See Barry Fell, *America, B.C.*)

69. The behavior of modern terrorists, in particular the willingness to die for what is usually a rather futile cause or demand, is a gruesome practical example of this viewpoint in the world today.

Glossary

SANSKRIT TERMS

Adwaite Vedanta. The non-dualist Truth; one of the six orthodox schools of Indian philosophy. This doctrine holds that Brahman is eternally unchanged and contains within "his" nature *maya,* or the eternal fiction of the manifestations of infinite possible realities.

Aham. The primary sense of "I," prior to the conception of other (see *Idam*). One of the greatest maxims of Gyana Yoga is the combined mantra *Aham Brahmasmi, Tat twam asi*—I am Brahman (the eternal Immense), Thou art That. (See Exodus: "I Am that I Am, go therefore and say to Pharaoh, 'I Am sent me.' ")

Ashtanga Yoga. The eight-limbed yoga codified by Patanjali. The limbs are: (1)*Yama*—abstention from malice, lying, coveting, acceptance of gifts, etc., and the control of the hidden organ of generation. The latter refers to the desire body, not, as generally interpreted, the sexual organ; (2)*Niyama*—observances; happiness for the happy, joy for the meritorious, indifference to evil, compassion for the sufferers; (3)*Asana*—literally, seat or the ability to sit for a long time; also refers to many other postures which help in the development of a balanced body. (4)*Pranayama*—literally, control of energy but taught as breathing exercises; (5)*Pratyahara*—withdrawal of the senses from their objects. This is often understood as a trance state, but more realistically it is the process of producing *Teh* or Virtue by controlling the inner needs (called the Indriyas or the gods of the senses); (6)*Dharana*—focused attention or one-pointed attention, often incorrectly translated as concentration. (7) *Dhyana*—contemplation; pondering the object of one-pointed attention; and (8)*Samadhi*—concentrated in concentration; seven levels of ever deeper concentration leading to *nirvikalpa samadhi,* or the seedless samadhi (concentration without an object of concentration).

Atman. The "real I" that is the root experience of individualized being. That which is experienced in deep meditation when the yogi truly enters the silence and experiences his nature as the individualized Absolute. Many believe that this is the ultimate experience sought by yogis, but it is not true.

Siddhartha expressed this to Gotama in the book *Siddhartha* by Herman Hesse. When Gotama had explained the path toward the Atman that he was teaching, Siddhartha bowed and departed saying to his companion that he'd had that experience since he was a boy and sought beyond.

Bhakti. Worship; the yoga of devotion in which the emotional nature is brought into harmony with the universal Truth. My Nada Yoga master, Swami Nada Brahmananda, saw his practice as worship; he said that he was the only swami in Sivananda's ashram in the Himalayas who had no books in his room. He worshiped and meditated through devotional music.

Bharata dharma. Bharata is the name for India long before her European contacts. Mahabharata refers to the great (*maha*) epic of Indian history. *Dharma* literally means "what holds together"; it often refers to the natural order or to one's specific duties. The Bharata dharma refers to the six great philosophical levels of Indian Philosophy, starting with basic materialism, through religious dualism, yogic dualism, and finally non-dualism, or Adwaite Vedanta.

Bhu loka. The Earth plane; the level of man's present manifestation world. Above are various heavens; below are various hells. We are in the middle.

Brahma. The Creator. One of the three primary forces, along with Vishnu, the sustainer (of the manifest world or illusion), and Shiva, the destroyer (of illusion).

Brahman. The Immense; the Absolute Uncreated Being.

Gyana Yoga. The yoga of self-knowledge. The stages are straightforward. Hear the Truth (Adwaite Vedanta) from a conscious source. Question and then ponder the Truth until there is no doubt. Meditate on the Truth, through negation of all that is not the Self (Is the Self the body? *Neti, neti,* or "not this, not this"; Is the Self the soul? *Neti, neti!* Is the Self Brahma? *Neti, neti,* and so on) until there is nothing left.

Idam. The "other" in the creation process. Shiva knows himself, *Aham.* He conceives of other, *Idam.* This is the beginning.

Ishwara. Literally, Lord or God. From the dualistic position, Ishwara is a special being which never enters into the world process, but waits for yogis to call upon him. He helps them attain higher states; his name is *OM* (*AUM*).

Iso-upanishad. One of most important of the ten major Upanishads. This work was translated by Swami Bhaktivedanta (truth from worship) as a religious document teaching the worship of Krishna. John Woodroofe's translation, which was done with the assistance of an unnamed Tantric scholar, is a true esoteric text.

Karma. The law of cause and effect. This law operates on the spiritual plane and therefore is not bound to linear chronological time. Also, the sum of the incomplete effects yet to occur.

Kundalini. The energy of the goddess, Shakti, which descends and creates all the worlds. It settles in the lowest manifestation and awaits stimulation to return to the source. Each yogi must, in one way or another, undergo the transformation of the Kundalini by reabsorption of the energy of the manifestation worlds or chakras.

Lila. Literally, divine play. The creative manifestation of God, also called *maya.*

Maya. The eternal fiction of infinite possible manifestations of the nature of the Absolute (Adwaite Vedanta).

Mudra. Asana (posture) that produces an activation of energy in the system. Term also refers to mystical hand gestures, sometimes spontaneous in certain forms of yoga. This can refer as well to burnt rice (one of the five forbidden things consumed in the rare Tantric ritual of the *virasadhaka*—the seeker who has control over very subtle energies and is brave as a warrior).

Nada Yoga. The yoga of sound. It includes the chanting of mantras to activate energy in the system, as well as the chanting of *bhajans,* or devotional songs with very complex scale (*raga*) and drum rhythm (*tala*) patterns, which build from comfortably slow to incredible speeds.

Nirguna Brahman. The Absolute without any attributes. The ultimate Reality.

Nirvikalpa Samadhi. The seedless samadhi; concentration without an object of concentration.

Niyama. The second of the eight practices of Ashtanga Yoga—the observances.

OM. The mystic syllable (Pranava), which is the name of Ishwara. This is written in Sanskrit as the three letters, A, U, and M. When used in meditation, the mouth is opened rather wide, and rounded. The tongue is drawn back, making a flat A sound. As the sound continues, the mouth is slowly closed, while the tongue gradually relaxes and moves forward to touch the back of the teeth. The elongated humming sound continues until no air is left. The sound procedes from the lower *tan tien* (A), then the middle *tan tien* (U), and finally vibrates at the upper *tan tien* (M).

Pranamaya Kosha. Literally, the sheath (*kosha*) in the form (*maya*) of energy (*prana*). One of the five bodies of man.

Purusha. Conscious element. According to Yoga Philosophy, the basic creation is dualistic. The two elements are Purusha, the consciousness or witness of experience, and Prakriti, the potential manifestations that the Purusha experiences.

Saguna Brahman. The Absolute with the three attributes of existence, consciousness, and bliss.

Satchidananda. The three attributes of Saguna Brahman mentioned above; these manifest in the world as being, knowing, and feeling.

Shakti. The female (active) aspect of Deity, particularly stressed by the Shaivite philosophers (followers of the God Shiva).

Shiva. The fecund principle; the creative source. The destroyer of illusion.

Sunyata. The Void, Wu Chi; that which, when filled up with everything, still remains empty.

Tantra Shastra. The latest of the revealed texts of India. The Vedas taught high philosophical ideas, but with the deterioration of the human race in the Kali Yuga, Shiva, at the urging of Parvati (Shakti), taught a new set of practices which were to help modern man reach enlightenment. These texts have been maligned because of a deep misunderstanding and the equation of the whole of Tantra, which actually permeates Indian life, as much of the daily religious practices, purifications, and rituals, with some very rare and advanced techniques of the inner circle of initiates (see *mudra*).

Upanishads. Philosophical texts which explain, in a variety of ways, the path from dualism to monism. It is interesting that the Brahmana class, the priests, invariably go to the Khastrya, the warrior-kings, for knowledge of the Monistic truth.

Vishnu. The sustainer of the Indian trilogy. Krishna is one of the avatars of Vishnu, the incarnations of divine love that are manifest to help mankind in times of extreme duress. This is in keeping with the role of sustainer of the illusion. The tenth avatar is yet to come.

Yama. The first set of formal practices of the eight-limbed yoga: restraint. It is also the name for the God of Death.

CHINESE TERMS

Chang San-feng. Legendary founder of T'ai Chi Chuan who lived in the thirteenth century; author of the *T'ai Chi Chuan Ching.*

Chi. Limit. The extreme condition, at which point a reversal takes place.

Ch'i. Will to action. The Demiurge underlying creation.

Du (Du Mai or *Du Mo).* The extraordinary channel that runs along the midline of the front of the body. It is called the Conception Vessel in English.

Hsing I Chuan. Literally, Mind Fist. One of the three classical inner schools.

Kung Fu. Achievement of skill or technique.

Kung Fu Tze (or Tzu). The "philosopher of right action," (Confu-cious), who codified the traditional value systems found in most oriental cultures.

Lao Tze (or Tzu). The "ancient philosopher"; source of fundamental Taoist thought and author of the *Tao Teh Ching.*

Li. The Idea, notion, or underlying reason, which activates an occurrence.

Moo Duk Kwan Tang Soo Do. A Korean style of Karate, which has strong Chinese influences. It translates as "the school of the virtuous warrior of the Art of Tang Dynasty hands."

Nei Chia. Inner schools of the martial arts concerned with the development of Qi.

Pa Kua Chang. Literally, eight-trigram palm. One of the three traditional inner schools of the martial arts.

Po. The animal soul, which resides in the lungs according to Chinese medical philosophy.

Qi. Energy/matter; the stuff of which the manifest universe is made. More particularly, invisible energies which can be used in healing and in martial arts.

Qi Kung. Exercises for the development and control of Qi. There are several forms of Qi Kung, some concerned with health, others with martial arts power or even magic.

Ren (Ren Mai or *Ren Mo).* The extraordinary channel that runs along the midline of the back and controls all Yang channels. In English it is called the Governing Vessel.

Shen. The heart or emotional center. The human soul which resides in the heart in Chinese medical philosophy.

T'ai Chi Chuan. Literally, the Great Limit Fist. One of the three classical inner schools of the martial arts.

Tan Tien. Literally, the field of pills. The center in which the psychic energies are conserved and transformed. In T'ai Chi Chuan, we are concerned with the opening and development of the lower *tan tien* and the circulation of Qi. Qi Kung evolves that circulation and works with the opening of the middle and upper *tan tien.*

Wang Shung Yueh. Fifteenth-century author of the two T'ai Chi Chuan classics, *The Mental Elucidation of the Thirteen Postures* and *The T'ai Chi Chuan Treatise,* quoted in this book.

Wing Tsun Kung Fu. A style of Kung Fu created by the Buddhist Nun Ng and taught to a young girl named Wing Chun (Tsun). This style is considered to be the first departure from the traditional methods of fighting in formal patterns. Bridge Hands, in which the arms only are used to attack and defend, is often practiced; this is first done in complex pre-arranged patterns, followed by a free form style.

Wu Chi. The Void or nothingness. A concept that describes the primordial state of the universe from which T'ai Chi arises.

Wu Chia. Martial arts schools concerned with the development of external power or *ching.*

Wu Tang. A famous mountain, also called Shao Lin.

Yung Chuan. Literally, bubbling spring. The first point on the Kidney meridian, located on the midline of the ball of the foot; point where the root is most powerful.

ENGLISH TERMS

Ancestral Qi. Qi that is built in the chest center by proper living and concomitant breath control exercises. It is inappropriately named, since the term implies that it is the "Qi of Prior Heaven," which is the fundamental life-sustaining Qi. With proper posture, exercise, and lifestyle, it can, however, increase to a point where it will convert to Qi of Prior Heaven. Qi Kung facilitates this process.

Bridge Hands. An exercise in Kung Fu which is akin to Push Hands in T'ai Chi Chuan. Practitioners slowly interact with their arms in attack and defense, maintaining continous contact with the opponent's arm. This exercise gradually increases in speed and complexity.

Cat Stance. A common martial arts stance in which the front foot point's forward and the rear foot, which bears most of the weight, is perpendicular to the front foot. Both legs are well bent. There are many variations of this stance.

Free Sparring. A developmental martial arts skill in which the practitioners attack and defend as if actually fighting, while executing controlled focused blows which fall just short of contact with the opponent.

Microcosmic Orbit. Energy circulation through the external pathways of the Acupuncture channels.

Push Hands. Slang for Joint Hands exercises in T'ai Chi Chuan. A kind of sparring in which partners stand facing each other and, without moving their feet, attempt to unbalance each other using minimum strength. A method of learning to sense energy.

MEDICAL TERMS

Abdomen—portion of trunk located between the chest and pelvis.

Abduct—to draw away from the midline of the body or one of its parts.

Abductor—a muscle that draws away from the midline of the body.

Acetabulum—the rounded cavity on the external surface of the hip bone that receives the head of the femur.

Achilles' tendon—the tendon of the gastrocnemius and soleus muscles of the leg that attaches to the calcaneus (heel bone).

Adduct—to draw towards the midline of the body or one of its parts.

Adductor—a muscle that draws towards the midline of the body or to a common center.

Adductor magnus—largest and deepest muscle of the adductor group, located on medial aspect of the thigh.

> *origin:* ischial tuberosity and pubic bone
> *insertion:* posterior shaft of femur and adductor tubercle of femur
> *action:* adduct thigh, assist flexion and extension of thigh

Adductor longus—longest and most superficial muscle of the adductor group located on medial aspect of the thigh.

> *origin:* anterior pubic bone
> *insertion:* posterior shaft of femur
> *action:* adduct thigh, assist flexion and medial rotation of thigh

Adductor brevis—located deep to adductor longus, shortest muscle of adductor group located on medial aspect of the thigh.

> *origin:* anterior pubic bone
> *insertion:* posterior shaft of femur
> *action:* adduct thigh, assist flexion and medial rotation of thigh

Anterior—before or in front of; ventral.

Arthritis—any inflammation of a joint, usually accompanied by pain, swelling, and frequently changes in structure.

Articulation—the place of union between two or more bones; a joint.

Bicep femoris—lateral muscle of the hamstring group located on the posterior/lateral aspect of the thigh.

> *origin:* ischial tuberosity, posterior shaft of femur
> *insertion:* proximal femur
> *action:* extends the hip, flexes the knee, laterally rotates the knee

Buttocks—the external prominences posterior to the hips, formed by the gluteal muscles and underlying structures.

Calcaneo-fibular ligament—a ligament of the lateral aspect of the ankle joint that connects the calcaneus (heel bone) to the fibula (lateral leg bone).

Calcaneus—heel bone.

Calf muscles—group of muscles located on the posterior aspect of the lower leg; gastrocnemius, soleus, and plantaris muscles.

Cervical—pertaining to or in the region of the neck.

Clavicle—collar bone.

Coccyx—small bone at the base of the spinal column formed by four fused vertebra; tail-bone.

Collateral ligaments of knee—two ligaments of the knee: the medial ligament passing from the medial condyle of the femur to the medial condyle of the tibia; the lateral passing from the lateral condyle of the femur to the head of the fibula.

Cruciate ligaments of knee—two ligaments of the knee: the anterior passing from the tibia to the lateral condyle of the femur; the posterior passing from the tibia to the medial condyle of the femur.

Deep lateral rotators—deep muscles of the gluteal region that extend from the sacrum and hip to the femur and all act to laterally rotate the thigh. This group includes: piriformis, gemellus superior and inferior, obturator internus and externus and quadratus femoris.

Deltoid—this muscle gives the shoulder its rounded contour.

  origin: lateral clavicle, acromion process and spine of scapula
  insertion: lateral shaft of humerus
  action: primary abductor of the arm; flexes, extends and rotates the arm

Dorsal—pertaining to the back, posterior; opposite of anterior or ventral.

Dorsiflexion—flexion of the foot at the ankle joint causing a decrease in the angle between the anterior surface of the articulating bones, i.e., in order to walk on one's heels the foot must be dorsiflexed at the ankle; opposite of plantarflexion.

Erector spinae—a large muscle lying on either side of the vertebral column extending from the sacrum to the head; also called sacrospinalis.

  origin: sacrum, ilium, lumbar vertebra, lower ribs
  insertion: upper ribs, thoracic and cervical vertebra, skull
  action: extend, laterally flex and rotate the vertebral column

Evert—to turn outward, i.e., movement of the sole of the foot outward (laterally) at the ankle.

Extension—a movement that brings the members of a limb into or towards a straight condition; opposite of flexion.

Extensor digitorum brevis—small muscle located on the dorsum (top) of the foot.

  origin: calcaneus
  insertion: phalanges of the toes
  action: assists in extension of the toes

Extensor digitorum longus—deep muscle of the anterior lateral leg.

  origin: tibia and fibula
  insertion: phalanges of toes
  action: extend toes, assist dorsiflexion of ankle

Extensor hallicus longus—deep muscle of the anterior lateral leg.

origin: fibula
insertion: base of great toe
action: extend great toe, assist dorsiflexion of ankle

External malleolus—bony prominence on the lateral aspect of the ankle; distal end of the fibula.

Facet joints of spine—small posterior joints of the spine located on either side of the spinous processes of the vertebra.

Femur—thigh bone; longest and strongest bone of the body.

Fibula—outer (lateral) and smaller bone of the lower leg.

Flexion—act of bending, or condition of being bent, in contrast to extension.

Gastrocnemius—most superficial of the calf muscles

origin: lower femur
insertion: calcaneus (Achille's tendon)
action: plantar flex ankle, assist flexion of the knee

Gluteus maximus—largest and most superficial muscle of the buttock.

origin: sacrum and ilium
insertions: femur and iliotibial tract
action: extend and laterally rotate thigh

Gluteus medius—deep to the gluteus maximus.

origin: ilium
insertion: femur
action: abduct and medially rotate thigh

Gluteus minimus—deep to gluteus medius.

origin: ilium
insertion: femur
action: abduct and medially rotate thigh

Gracilis—the most superficial of the adductor muscles located on the medial aspect of the thigh. The focus of the Lymph Rub is deep massage of the lymph vessels along the belly of this muscle.

origin: pubic bone
insertion: proximal tibia
action: adduct thigh; assist flexion and medial rotation of knee

Groin—the depression between the thigh and trunk formed by the origins of the adductor muscles to the pubic bone.

Hamstrings—three muscles on the posterior aspect of the thigh: biceps femoris, semitendinosus, semimembranosus.

Humerus—bone of the upper arm.

Hyoid muscles—a group of muscles that insert into the hyoid bone located on the anterior aspect of the neck. These muscles control swallowing.

Hyperextension—extreme or abnormal extension.

Ilium—superior and widest part of the pelvic bone. The upper part of the ilium is commonly referred to as the waist.

Iliofemoral ligament—ligament of the anterior/superior hip joint, which extends from the ilium to the femur.

Iliopsoas—the compound iliacus and psoas muscles.

> *origin:* lumbar vertebra and ilium
> *insertion:* femur
> *action:* flexes, abducts, and laterally rotates thigh

Iliotibial tract—a thick broad band of connective tissue extending from the ilium to the tibia on the lateral aspect of the thigh.

Inguinal—see groin.

Innominate—pelvic or hip bone consisting of ilium, ischium, and pubis. United with the sacrum and coccyx by ligaments to form the pelvis.

Invert—to turn inward, i.e., movement of the sole of the foot inward (medially) at the ankle.

Interspinous—between the spinous processes of the vertebra.

Intervertebral—between the vertebra.

Ischial tuberosity—large prominence on the inferior aspect of the pelvic bone that supports weight while sitting.

Ischiofemoral ligament—ligament of the posterior/inferior hip joint, which extends from the acetabulum to the femur.

Lateral—to the side or pertaining to the side; opposite of medial.

Latissimus dorsi—widest and most superficial muscle of the lower back.

> *origin:* ilium, sacrum, lower thoracic and lumbar vertebra
> *insertion:* anterior humerus
> *action:* extension, adduction and medial rotation of humerus, and hyperextension of the arm. Through its action on the arm, can also depress the shoulder

Ligament—dense connective tissue that attaches bone to bone.

Ligamentum flava—elastic ligament located between the vertebra.

Ligamentum teres—a round ligament that connects the head of the femur with the acetabulum.

Linea alba—the white line of connective tissue along the midline of the abdomen running from the sternum (breast bone) to the pubis.

Longitudinal ligaments—two ligaments of the vertebral column: the anterior runs along the front of the vertebra, the posterior runs within the spinal canal, anterior to the spinal cord.

Lumbar—pertaining to the lower back, the area between the thorax and pelvis; loin.

Lymphatic system—all structures involved in the conveyance of lymph from the tisssues to the bloodstream. The "sewer system" of the body.

Medial—nearer the midline of the body; opposite of lateral.

Nuchal ligament—an elastic ligament located between the spinous processes of the cervical vertebra.

Oncological—pertaining to tumors.

Orbital ridge of the eye—the bony edge of the eye socket.

Patella—kneecap.

Pectineus—uppermost muscle of the medial thigh muscles.

> *origin:* pubic bone

insertion: posterior femur

action: flexes thigh, assists adduction and medial rotation of thigh

Pelvis—the bony basin-shaped structure formed by the hip, sacrum, coccyx, and the ligaments supporting them. The structure serves as a support for the vertebral column and for articulation with the lower limbs.

Perineum—the pelvic floor; the region between the anus and the genital.

Peroneus brevis—shortest of the peroneal muscles.

origin: lateral fibula

insertion: lateral edge of foot

action: everts foot, assists in plantarflexion of foot

Peroneus longus—longest of the peroneal muscles, its tendon passes under the foot to form a stirrup with the tendon of the tibialis anterior.

origin: lateral fibula

insertion: inferior aspect of the medial edge of foot

action: everts foot, assists in plantarflexion of foot

Pertoneus tertius—the most anterior of the peroneal muscles.

origin: anterior fibula

insertion: lateral edge of foot

action: everts foot, assists in dorsiflexion of foot

Plantarflexion—extension of the foot at the ankle, i.e., to walk on one's toes the foot must be plantarflexed; opposite of dorsiflex.

Plantaris—a long slim muscle of the calf located between the gastrocnemius and the soleus.

origin: lateral femur

insertion: calcaneus (Achille's tendon)

action: assists plantarflexion of ankle and flexion of the knee

Platysma—most superficial muscle on the anterior aspect of the neck.

origin: connective tissue of the chest and shoulder

insertion: lower jaw and skin of lower face

action: tenses skin of neck and depresses jaw

Popliteus—deepest muscle at the back of the knee.

origin: lateral femur

insertion: posterior tibia

action: initiates knee flexion by medial rotation of tibia

Posterior—nearer to or at the back of the body; dorsal.

Proximal—nearer to the point of origin; nearer the attachment of an extremity to the trunk or a structure.

Pubis—the lower anterior part of the pelvic bone.

Pubofemoral ligament—ligament of the anterior/inferior hip joint, which extends from the pubis to the femur.

Pyramidalis—small triangular muscle of the lower abdominal wall.

origin: pubic bone

insertion: linea alba

action: tightens lower abdominal wall

Quadratus lumborum—deep muscle of the posterior abdominal wall.

origin: ilium
insertion: 12th rib, lumbar vertebra
action: lateral flexion of trunk or raises hip

Quadriceps femoris—four large muscles of the anterior thigh which act to extend the knee: rectus femoris, vastus medialis, vastus lateralis, vastus intermedius.

Rectus abdominis—most prominent muscle on the anterior abdominal wall.

origin: pubis
insertion: lower rib cage
action: flexes trunk, compresses abdominal contents

Rheumatism—a general term for acute and chronic conditions characterized by inflammation, soreness, and stiffness of muscles and pain in joints and associated structures.

Rhomboids—muscle deep to the trapezius in the upper back.

origin: upper thoracic vertebra
insertion: medial border of scapula
action: retracts (adducts) and rotates scapula

Sacroiliac joint—the articulation betwen the pelvis and sacrum.

Sacrum—a triangular bone formed by the union of five sacral vertebrae, positioned between the fifth lumbar vertebra and the coccyx and between the two hip bones. The sacrum serves as a strong foundation for the pelvic girdle.

Sartorius—the most superficial muscle of the anterior thigh and the longest muscle in the body.

origin: ilium
insertion: medial tibia
action: assists flexion, abducts and laterally rotates thigh, assists flexion and medially rotates knee

Scapula—large flat triangular bone that forms the posterior part of the shoulder; shoulder blade.

Semimembranosus—the most medial of the hamstring muscles.

origin: ischial tuberosity
insertion: posterior tibia
action: flexes knee, extends thigh, medially rotates flexed knee

Semitendinosus—located between the semimembranosus and bicep femoris.

origin: ischial tuberosity
insertion: anterior tibia
action: flexes knee, extends thigh, medially rotates flexed knee

Serratus anterior—located under the scapula and on the lateral wall of the thorax.

origin: upper ribs
insertion: medial border of scapula
action: protracts (abducts) scapula, rotates scapula, stabilizes scapula against chest wall

Splenius capitis and cervicis—muscles located deep to the upper trapezius on the posterior aspect of the neck.

origin: upper thoracic and lower cervical vertebra
insertion: upper cervical vertebra and skull
action: extend and rotate neck

Spinous process—prominence at posterior part of each vertebra.

Talocalcaneal ligaments—two ligaments located medially and laterally between the talus and calcaneus bones.

Talofibular ligaments—two ligaments located anteriorly and posteriorly on the lateral aspect of the ankle joint between the talus and the fibula.

Talus—the ankle bone articulating with the tibia, fibula, and calcaneus.

Tendon—dense connective tissue that attaches muscle to bone.

Tensor fascia lata—small muscle of the lateral hip.

> *origin:* ilium
> *insertion:* iliotibial tract
> *action:* stabilizes knee during walking, assists abduction, medial rotation, flexion of the thigh, and extension of the knee

Thoracic—pertaining to the chest.

Tibia—inner (medial) and larger bone of the lower leg.

Tibialis anterior—the most superficial muscle on the anterior leg.

> *origin:* lateral tibia
> *insertion:* medial edge of foot
> *action:* primary dorsiflexor of foot, inverts foot

Trapezius—large superficial triangular muscle of the posterior neck and shoulders that consists of three parts—upper, middle, and lower trapezius.

> *origin:* skull, spinous processes of cervical and thoracic vertebra
> *insertion:* upper—clavicle and upper scapula
> middle—ridge across posterior scapula
> lower—mid-medial border of scapula
> *action:* upper—raises and rotates scapula
> middle—retracts (adducts) scapula
> lower—depresses and rotates scapula

Transversospinalis muscle group—small muscles of the spine which act to extend and rotate the vertebral column. These muscles lie deep to the erector spinae and are found in order from superficial to deep: semispinalis, multifidus, rotatores, interspinales, intertransversarii.

Urogenital system—pertinent to the urinary and reproductive organs.

Suggested Readings

BOOKS ON T'AI CHI CHUAN AND HARA

Cheng Man-Ch'ing and Robert W. Smith. *T'ai Chi*. Rutland, VT: Charles E. Tuttle, 1967.

Da Liu. *T'ai Chi Chuan and I Ching*. New York: Harper & Row, 1950.

Durckheim, Karlfried. *Hara*. New York: Weiser, 1962.

Huang Wen-Shan. *Fundamentals of T'ai Chi Chuan*. Hong Kong: South Sky Book Co., 1974.

Jou, Tsung Hwa. *The Tao of T'ai Chi Chuan*. Rutland, VT: Charles E. Tuttle, 1980.

Lee Ying-Arng. *Lee's Modified T'ai Chi for Health*. Honolulu, HI: McLisa Enterprises, 1968.

Yearning K. Chen. *T'ai Chi Chuan: It's Effects and Practical Application*. Los Angeles: O'hara Publications, 1979.

BOOKS ON ESOTERIC PHILOSOPHY

Aurelius, Marcus. *Meditations*. Translated by A.S.L. Farquharson. New York: Dutton, 1961.

Lao-Tzu. *Tao Teh Ching*. Edited by Gia-fu Feng and translated by Jane English. New York: Knopf, 1974.

Lu, K'uan Yu. *Taoist Yoga*. York Beach, Maine: Weiser, 1984.

Miyamoto, Musashi. *A Book of Five Rings*. Translated by Victor Harris. Woodstock, NY: Overlook Press, 1980.

Ouspensky, P.D. *Tertium Organum*. New York: Knopf, 1947.

———. *A New Model of the Universe*. New York: Knopf, 1949.

———. *In Search of the Miraculous.* New York: Harcourt Brace Jovanovich, 1965.

Ryle, Gilbert. *The Concept of Mind.* New York: Hutchinson's University Library, 1949.

Sohn, Robert C. *On Willingness To Be Wrong.* Manhasset, NY: Sivamokshananda Press, 1978.

————. *On Transcendental Aim.* Manhasset, NY: Sivamokshananda Press, 1979.

————. *The Reality of Living Yoga.* Manhasset, NY: Sivamokshananda Press, 1980.

Woods, Christopher. *The Yoga System of Patanjali.* New Delhi: Motilal Banarsidass, 1972.

BOOKS ON ANCIENT HISTORY

Chiera, Edward. *They Wrote on Clay.* Chicago: University of Chicago Press, 1938.

Coe, Michael D. *The Maya.* New York: Thames & Hudson, 1987.

Fell, Barry. *America, BC: Ancient Settlers in the New World.* New York: Simon & Schuster, 1976.

Gaur, Albertine. *A History of Writing.* New York: Scribner, 1984.

Heidel, Alexander. *The Gilgamesh Epic and Old Testament Parallels.* Chicago: University of Chicago Press, 1949.

Jaynes, Julian. *The Origin of Consciousness in the Breakdown of the Bicameral Mind.* Boston: Houghton Mifflin, 1976.

Norman, James, *Ancestral Voices: Decoding Ancient Languages.* New York: Four Winds Press, 1975.

Pope, Maurice. *The Story of Archaeological Decipherment: From Egyptian Hieroglyphis to Linear B.* New York: Scribner, 1975.

White, J.E. Manchip. *Ancient Egypt.* New York: Dover, 1970.

Woolley, C. Leonard, *The Sumerians.* New York: Norton, 1965.

BOOKS ON MEDICINE AND SCIENCE

Barral, Jean-Pierre and Pierre Mercier. *Visceral Manipulation.* Seattle, WA: Eastland Press, 1988.

Darwin, Charles. *The Descent of Man.* Norwalk, CT: Easton Press, 1979.

Tompkins, Peter and Christopher Bird. *The Secret Life of Plants.* New York: Avon Books, 1973.

Sheldon, W. *The Varieties of Human Physique.* New York: Hafner, 1970.

————. *The Varieties of Human Temperment.* New York: Hafner, 1970.

Sohn, Tina. *Amma: The Ancient Art of Oriental Healing.* Rochester, VT: Healing Arts Press, 1988.

Zukav, Gary. *The Dancing Wu Li Masters: An Overview of the New Physics.* New York: Morrow, 1979.

Index

I would like to acknowledge the following people for their help in the creation of this book. Suṣhila Blackman for her astute editing. The Production Editor, Susan Davidson, for her calm and helpful manner. Johnnie W.C. Ng for the beautiful calligraphy. Mark Feinberg for his photography. Robert Young for posing in several photos. Joel Leibowitz for reading, questioning, rereading, and requestioning until the philosophical aspects of the text became comprehensible. Finally, Steven Schenkman for his help in creating the anatomical and physiological descriptions of the exercises.